THE DOCTOR'S GUIDE TO CRITICAL APPRAISAL

THIRD EDITION

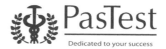

PasTest

Dedicated to your success

Dedicated to our son, Dilip, whose inquisitive nature reminds us that we should never stop asking questions.

THE DOCTOR'S GUIDE
TO CRITICAL APPRAISAL

THIRD EDITION

Dr Narinder Kaur Gosall

BSc (Hons) PhD

Director, Superego Cafe Limited

Dr Gurpal Singh Gosall

MA MB BChir MRCPsych

Consultant General Adult Psychiatrist,

Lancashire Care NHS Foundation Trust

Director, Superego Cafe Limited

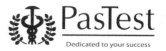

© 2012 PasTest Ltd

Egerton Court
Parkgate Estate
Knutsford
Cheshire WA16 8DX

Telephone: 01565 752000

First edition 2006, Second edition 2009, Third edition 2012

Reprinted October 2012

ISBN: 1 905635 818
ISBN: 978 1 905635 818
A catalogue record for this book is available from the British Library.

PasTest Revision Books and Intensive Courses

PasTest has been established in the field of undergraduate and postgraduate medical education since 1972, providing revision books and intensive study courses for doctors preparing for their professional examinations.

Books and courses are available for:

Medical undergraduates, MRCGP, MRCP Parts 1 and 2, MRCPCH Parts 1 and 2, MRCS, MRCOG Parts 1 and 2, DRCOG, DCH, FRCA, Dentistry.

For further details contact:

PasTest, Freepost, Knutsford, Cheshire, WA16 7BR

Tel: 01565 752000   **Fax: 01565 650264**

www.pastest.co.uk   **enquiries@pastest.co.uk**

Text prepared by Carnegie Book Production, Lancaster
Printed and bound by CPI Group (UK) Ltd, Croydon, CR0 4YY

CONTENTS

About the authors   vii
Introduction to the third edition   viii
Acknowledgements   ix

SECTION A – EVIDENCE-BASED MEDICINE   1

Introducing critical appraisal   3
Formulating a question   7
Search strategies   9
The journal   11
Organisation of the article   13

SECTION B – APPRAISING THE METHODOLOGY   15

Overview of methodology   17
The clinical question   18
Introducing study designs   22
Observational descriptive studies   24
Observational analytical studies   25
Experimental studies   30
Other types of study   36
Research pathway   40
Populations and samples   42
Bias   44
Confounding factors   49
Restriction   54
Matching   55
Randomisation   56
Concealed allocation   60
The placebo effect   62
Blinding   65
Endpoints   69
Validity   72
Reliability   74

SECTION C – INTERPRETING RESULTS   79

Basic statistical terms   81
Epidemiological data   82
Intention-to-treat analysis   86
Risks and odds   91

Types of data   100
Measuring data   102
Data distributions   105
Describing categorical data   108
Describing normally distributed data   109
Describing non-normally distributed data   113
Inferring population results from samples   117
Comparing samples – the null hypothesis   121
Comparing samples – statistical tests   129
Non-inferiority and equivalence trials   137
Correlation and regression   139
Systematic reviews and meta-analyses   145
Heterogeneity and homogeneity   151
Publication bias   155
Interim analysis   158

SECTION D – USING CHECKLISTS   **159**

Introduction to checklists   161
Aetiological studies   162
Diagnostic or screening studies   164
Treatment studies   173
Prognostic studies   175
Economic studies   179
Qualitative research   185
Guidelines   190

SECTION E – APPLICABILITY   **193**

The hierarchy of evidence   195
Critical thinking   198

SECTION F – CRITICAL APPRAISAL IN PRACTICE   **203**

Health information resources   205
Presenting at a journal club   209
Taking part in an audit meeting   212
Working with pharmaceutical representatives   214

Further reading   218
Answers to self-assessment exercises   221
A final thought   231
Index   232

Dr Narinder Kaur Gosall BSc (Hons) PhD

Director, Superego Cafe Limited

Narinder Gosall studied in Liverpool and gained a PhD in neuropathology after investigating the role of the phrenic nerve in sudden infant death syndrome and intrauterine growth retardation. After working as a university lecturer she joined the pharmaceutical industry. She worked in a variety of roles, including as a Medical Liaison Executive and as a Clinical Effectiveness Consultant for Pfizer Limited. She has extensive experience in teaching critical appraisal skills to healthcare professionals and is an international speaker on the subject. She is the editor of the online course at www.criticalappraisal.com.

Dr Gurpal Singh Gosall MA MB BChir MRCPsych

Consultant General Adult Psychiatrist, Lancashire Care NHS Foundation Trust

Director, Superego Cafe Limited

Gurpal Gosall studied medicine at the University of Cambridge and Guy's and St Thomas's Hospitals, London. He worked as a Senior House Officer in Psychiatry in Leeds before taking up a post as Specialist Registrar in the North West. He now works as a Consultant Psychiatrist, looking after patients in the Psychiatric Intensive Care Units at the Royal Blackburn Hospital and Burnley General Hospital. He has a long-standing interest in teaching and runs a popular website for psychiatrists, Superego Cafe, at www.superego-cafe.com.

INTRODUCTION TO THE THIRD EDITION

Learning the skill of critical appraisal is like learning a foreign language – wherever you start, you come across unfamiliar words and concepts. However, persistence pays off and, like speaking a foreign language, the earlier it is mastered and the more it is used, the easier critical appraisal becomes.

Critical appraisal skills are now as much a part of the clinician's armoury as the ability to diagnose conditions and prescribe treatments. Critical appraisal skills allow clinicians to prioritise evidence that can improve outcomes. Such is the importance of acquiring these skills that critical appraisal is now routinely tested in medical, dental and nursing exams.

We wrote the first edition of this book 6 years ago to explain critical appraisal to the busy clinician. Our aim has always been for the book to be the one-stop solution for all clinicians. Based on our teaching experience, we took a unique back-to-basics approach that provided a logical and comprehensive review of the subject. This new edition expands on the last edition with updated information, new chapters and more help with difficult topics.

We hope that by reading this book you will start reading and appraising clinical papers with more confidence. The language of evidence-based medicine is not as foreign as you might think.

NKG, GSG

2012

ACKNOWLEDGEMENTS

We would like to express our thanks to Cathy Dickens (Senior Commissioning Editor), Fiona Power (Technical Editor), Sarah Price (Proof-reader), Lucy Frontani (Typesetter) and the PasTest team for their help and support with this book. Thanks also to Elizabeth Kerr, formerly of PasTest, who worked on the first edition.

We thank our teachers and colleagues for generously sharing their knowledge and for providing guidance. We are also indebted to all the doctors, dentists, nurses, psychologists, pharmacists, researchers and other healthcare professionals who have attended our critical appraisal courses and provided us with comments and helpful suggestions about our teaching materials.

We would like to express our gratitude to our families, who inspired us and gave us unconditional support during the writing of this book. In addition, a special thank you goes to Guj for his constant belief and encouragement during our endeavours.

January 2012

SECTION A

EVIDENCE-BASED MEDICINE

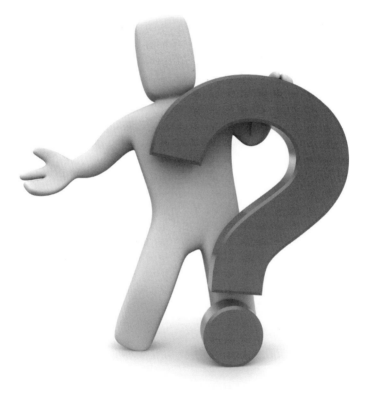

Scenario 1

Dr Jones was annoyed. Six months ago, he was given a clinical paper by a pharmaceutical sales representative about a new treatment for high blood pressure. The results of the trial were certainly impressive. On the basis of the evidence presented, he prescribed the new tablet to all his hypertensive patients. Instead of the expected finding that 4/5 patients would have lowered blood pressure, only 1/10 patients improved. He decided to present the article at the hospital journal club, as he couldn't see where in the study the mistake lay. He then hoped to confront the sales representative for wasting his time and the hospital's money.

Every year, thousands of clinical papers are published in the medical press. The vast range of topics reflects the sheer complexity of the human body, with studies all fighting for our attention. Separating the wheat from the chaff is a daunting task for doctors, many of whom have to rely on others for expert guidance.

In 1972, the publication of Archie Cochrane's *Effectiveness and efficiency: random reflections on health services*[1] made doctors realise how unaware they were of the effects of healthcare. Archie Cochrane, a British epidemiologist, went on to set up the Cochrane Collaboration in 1992. It is now an international organisation, committed to producing and disseminating systematic reviews of healthcare interventions. Bodies such as the Cochrane Collaboration have made the lives of doctors much easier, but the skill of evaluating evidence should be in the arsenal of every doctor.

Evidence-based medicine

Evidence-based medicine is the phrase used to describe the process of practising medicine based on a combination of the best available research evidence, our clinical expertise and patient values. As such, evidence-based medicine has had a tremendous impact on improving healthcare outcomes since its widespread adoption in the early 1990s.

The most widely quoted definition of evidence-based medicine is that it is *'the conscientious, explicit and judicious use of current best evidence in making*

1   Cochrane AL. *Effectiveness and Efficiency: Random Reflections on Health Services.* London, Royal Society of Medicine Press, 1999.

decisions about the care of the individual patient[1]. The practice of evidence-based medicine consists of five steps, shown in **Table 1**.

	EVIDENCE-BASED MEDICINE – THE FIVE STEPS	
1	Question	Formulate a precise, structured clinical question about an aspect of patient management
2	Evidence	Search for the best evidence with which to answer the question
3	Critical appraisal	Evaluate the evidence, critically appraising the evidence for its validity, impact and applicability
4	Application	Apply the results to clinical practice, integrating the critical appraisal with clinical expertise and with patients' circumstances
5	Implementation and monitoring	Implement and monitor this process, evaluating the effectiveness and efficacy of the whole process, and identifying ways of improving them both for the future

Table 1 Evidence-based medicine – the five steps

Evidenced-based medicine begins with the formulation of a clinical question, such as *'What is the best treatment for carpal tunnel syndrome?'* This is followed by a search of the medical literature, looking for answers to the question. The evidence gathered is appraised and the recommendations from the best studies are applied to patients. The final step, which is often overlooked, is to monitor any changes and repeat the process.

Although evidence-based medicine has led to a more consistent and uniform approach to clinical practice, it does not mean that clinicians practise identically. Clinicians vary in their level of expertise, so not all the recommendations from clinical research can be followed. For example, the evidence might suggest that an intramuscular injection is the best treatment for a condition but the clinician might not have been trained to safely administer that treatment. In addition, patients differ in the interventions they find acceptable – some patients prefer not to have injections, for example. Finally, a lack of resources can also restrict the choices available, particularly for new and expensive interventions.

1   Sackett DL, Richardson WS, Rosenberg W, Haynes RB. *Evidence-based Medicine: How to Practise and Teach Evidence-based Medicine.* London, Churchill Livingstone, 1997.

Critical appraisal

In the process of evidence-based medicine, why do we need a step of critical appraisal? Why not take all results at face value and apply all the findings to clinical practice? The first reason is that there might be conflicting conclusions drawn from different studies. Secondly, real-life medicine rarely follows the restrictive environments in which clinical trials take place. To apply, implement and monitor evidence, we need to ensure that the evidence we are looking at can be translated into our own clinical environment.

Critical appraisal is just one step in the process of evidence-based medicine. It allows doctors to assess the research they have found in their search and to decide which research evidence could have a clinically significant impact on their patients. Critical appraisal allows doctors to exclude research that is too poorly designed to inform medical practice. By itself, critical appraisal does not lead to improved outcomes. It is only when the conclusions drawn from critically appraised studies are applied to everyday practice and monitored that the outcomes for patients improve.

Critical appraisal assesses the validity of the research and statistical techniques employed in studies and generates clinically useful information from them. It seeks to answer two major questions:

- Does the research have **internal validity** – to what extent does the study measure what it sets out to measure?
- Does the research have **external validity** – to what extent can the results from the study be generalised to a wider population?

As with most subjects in medicine, it is not possible to learn about critical appraisal without coming across jargon. Wherever we start, we will come across words and phrases we do not understand. In this book we try to explain critical appraisal in a logical and easy-to-remember way. Anything unfamiliar will be explained in due course.

Efficacy and effectiveness

Two words that are useful to define now are 'efficacy' and 'effectiveness'. These words are sometimes used interchangeably but they have different meanings and consequences in the context of evidence-based medicine.

Efficacy describes the impact of interventions under optimal (trial) conditions.

Effectiveness is a different but related concept, describing whether the interventions have the intended or expected effect under ordinary (clinical) circumstances.

Efficacy shows that internal validity is present. Effectiveness shows that external validity (generalisability) is present.

The contrast between efficacy and effectiveness studies was first highlighted in 1967 by Schwartz and Lellouch[1]. Efficacy studies usually have the aim of seeking regulatory approval for licensing. The interventions in such studies tend to be strictly controlled and compared with placebo interventions. The people taking part in such studies tend to be a selective 'eligible' population. In contrast, effectiveness studies tend to be undertaken for formulary approval. Dosing regimens are usually more flexible and are compared with interventions already being used. Almost anyone is eligible to enter such trials.

It is not always easy and straightforward to translate the results from clinical trials (efficacy data) to uncontrolled clinical settings (effectiveness data). The results achieved in everyday practice do not always mirror an intervention's published efficacy data and there are many reasons for this. The efficacy of an intervention is nearly always more impressive than its effectiveness.

Scenario 1 revisited

The journal club audience unanimously agreed that the double-blind randomised controlled trial was conducted to a high standard. The methodology, the analysis of the results and the conclusions drawn could not be criticised. When Dr Jones queried why his results were so different, the chairman of the journal club commented, 'My colleague needs to understand the difference between efficacy data and his effectiveness data. I assume his outpatient clinic and follow-up arrangements are not run to the exacting standards of a major international trial! May I suggest that, before criticising the work of others, he should perhaps read a book on critical appraisal?'

1   Schwartz D, Lellouch J. Explanatory and pragmatic attitudes in therapeutical trials. *Journal of Chronic Diseases* 1967, 20, 637–48.

FORMULATING A QUESTION

The first step in adopting an evidence-based medicine approach is to formulate a precise, structured clinical question about an aspect of patient management. Getting the right answer depends on asking the right question. Broad questions such as, 'How do I treat diabetes mellitus?' and 'What causes bowel cancer?' are easy to understand but return too many results on searching the medical literature.

PICO

The acronym 'PICO', explained in **Table 2**, can lead to a more focused search strategy. PICO phrases questions in a way that directs the search to relevant and precise answers.

P	Patient or Problem	Describe your patient and their problem
I	Intervention	Describe the main intervention, exposure, test or prognostic factor under consideration
C	Comparison	In the case of treatment, describe a comparative intervention (although a comparison is not always needed)
O	Outcomes	Describe what you hope to achieve, measure or affect

Table 2 Introducing PICO

For example, a doctor assesses a new patient presenting with depressive symptoms. The doctor decides to prescribe antidepressant medication. The patient is worried about side-effects and asks the doctor if there are any other treatment options. The doctor has heard that cognitive behavioural therapy has been used to treat depression. The doctor carries out a search of the medical literature using the PICO search strategy shown in **Table 3**.

P	Patient or Problem	In a man with depression...
I	Intervention	...is cognitive behavioural therapy...
C	Comparison	...compared with fluoxetine...
O	Outcomes	...better at improving depressive symptoms?

Table 3 An example of PICO

SEARCH STRATEGIES

By adopting a sensible search technique you can dramatically improve the outcome of a search. You might begin by formulating a PICO research question. This will enable you to perform a more structured search for the relevant information and will indicate where the information needs lie. Keywords, similar words or synonyms should then be identified, to search terms on the database.

When you start the search you want to ensure that the search is not too narrow – that is, that you get as many papers as possible to look at. This is done by **exploding your search**. This means that you can search for a keyword plus all the associated narrower terms simultaneously. As a result, all articles that have been indexed as narrow terms and that are listed below the broader term are included. If too many results are returned, you can refine the search and get more specific results – **focusing your search**. Filters can be used to increase the effectiveness of the search. Subheadings can be used alongside index terms to narrow the search. Indexers can assign keywords to an article. These words can also be weighted by labelling them as major headings. These are then used to represent the main concepts of an article. This can help focus the search even more.

Search engines are not normally case-sensitive – 'Diabetes' and 'diabetes' will return the same results. To search for a phrase, enclose it in **quotation marks** – 'treatment of diabetes mellitus' will only return items with that phrase, for example.

Boolean operators are used to combine together keywords and phrases in your search strategy:

- **AND** is used to link together different subjects. This is used when you are focusing your search and will retrieve fewer references. For example, 'diabetes' AND 'insulin inhalers' will return items containing both terms.

- **OR** is used to broaden your search. You would use OR to combine like subjects or synonyms. For example, 'diabetes' OR 'hyperglycaemia' will return items containing either term.

- **NOT** is used to exclude material from a search. For example, 'diabetes' NOT 'insipidus' will return items containing the first term and not the second.

Parentheses (nesting): This can be used to clarify relationships between search terms. For example, '(diabetes or hyperglycaemia)' AND 'inhalers' will return items containing either of the first two terms and the third.

Truncation: A **truncation** symbol at the end of a word returns any possible endings to that word. For example, 'cardio*' will return 'cardiology', 'cardiovascular' and 'cardiothoracic'. There are a variety of truncation symbols in use, including a question mark (?), an asterisk (*) and a plus sign (+).

Wild cards: A **wild card** symbol within a word will return the possible characters that can be substituted. For example, 'wom#n' will return 'woman' and 'women'. Common wild-card symbols include the hash (#) and the question mark (?).

Stemming: Most search engines will 'stem' search words. Stemming removes suffixes such as '-s', '-ing' and '-ed'. These variations are returned automatically when stem words are searched.

Thesaurus: This is used in some databases, such as MEDLINE, to help perform more effective searching. It is a controlled vocabulary and is used to index information from different journals. This is done by grouping related concepts under a single preferred term. As a result, all indexers use the same standard terms to describe a subject area, regardless of the term the author has chosen to use. It contains keywords, definitions of those keywords and cross-references between keywords. In healthcare, the National Library of Medicine uses a thesaurus called **Medical Subject Headings (MeSH)**. MeSH contains more than 17 000 terms. Each of these keywords represents a single concept appearing in the medical literature. For most MeSH terms, there will be broader, narrower and related terms to consider for selection. MeSH can also be used by the indexers in putting together entries for MEDLINE databases.

Synonyms: Search engines might expand searches by using a thesaurus to match search words to other words with the same meaning.

Plus (+) symbol: Use a **plus (+)** symbol before a term that must appear in the search results. For example, '+glucophage diabetes' will return items that include the Glucophage brand name and diabetes rather than the generic name metformin.

Sources of information

There is no single definitive source of medical information. A comprehensive search strategy will use a number of different sources to ensure that all relevant material is retrieved. Some popular sources are listed on pages 205–208.

Not all journals are equal. Some journals are more prestigious than others. There can be many reasons for such prestige, including a long history in publishing, affiliation with an important medical organisation or a reputation for publishing important research. It is important to know which journal an article was published in – but remember, even the best journals sometimes publish poor articles and good papers can appear in the less prestigious journals.

Peer-reviewed journals

A **peer-reviewed** journal is a publication that requires each submitted article to be independently examined by a panel of experts, who are non-editorial staff of the journal. To be considered for publication, articles need to be approved by the majority of peers. The process is usually anonymous, with the authors not knowing the identities of the peer reviewers. In double-blind peer review, neither the author nor the reviewers know the others' identities. Anonymity aids the feedback process.

The peer-review process forces authors to meet certain standards laid down by researchers and experts in that field. Peer review makes it more likely that mistakes or flaws in research are detected before publication. As a result of this quality assurance, peer-reviewed journals are regarded in greater esteem than non-peer-reviewed journals.

There are disadvantages to the peer-review process, however. Firstly, it adds a delay between the submission of an article and its publication. Secondly, the peer reviewers might guess the identity of the author(s), particularly in small, specialised fields, impairing the objectivity of their assessments. Thirdly, revolutionary or unpopular conclusions can face opposition within the peer-review process, leading to preservation of the status quo. Finally, it is worth remembering that peer review does not guarantee that errors will not appear in the finished article or that fraudulent research will not be published.

Journal impact factor

A high number of citations implies that a journal is found to be useful to others, suggesting that the research published in that journal is valuable. However, simply ranking a journal's importance by the number of times articles within that journal are cited by others would favour large journals over small journals and frequently issued journals over less frequently issued journals.

A **journal impact factor** provides a means of evaluating or comparing the performance of a journal relative to that of others in the same field. It ranks a journal's importance by the number of times articles within that journal are cited by others. Impact factors are calculated annually by Thomson Reuters (formerly known as the Institute for Scientific Information) and published in the *Journal Citation Report* (JCR).

The journal impact factor[1] is a measure of the frequency with which the average article in a journal has been cited in a particular year. The impact factor is the number of citations in the current year to articles published in the two previous years, divided by the total number of articles published in the two previous years. In 2011 the *New England Journal of Medicine* had an impact factor of 53.48 and the *British Medical Journal* had an impact factor of 13.471.

It is important to remember, in critical appraisal, that the journal impact factor cannot be used to assess the importance of any one article, as the impact factor is a property of the journal and is not specific to that article. Also, journal citation counts in JCR do not distinguish between letters, reviews or original research.

The **immediacy index** is another way from Thomson Reuters of evaluating journals. It measures how often articles published in a journal are cited within the same year. This is useful for comparing journals specialising in cutting-edge research.

A journal can improve its impact factor by improving accessibility to its articles and publicising them more widely. In recent years there have been significant improvements in web-based access to journals and now some journals publish research articles online before they appear in print. Many journals issue press releases highlighting research findings and send frequent email alerts to subscribers. A rise in the percentage of review articles published in a journal can also boost its impact factor. Review journals often occupy the first-ranked journal position in the JCR subject category listings.

---

1   *Journal Citation Report (JCR)*. Philadelphia, USA. Thomson Institute for Scientific Information, 2005. JCR provides quantitative tools for ranking, evaluating, categorising and comparing journals.

ORGANISATION OF THE ARTICLE

The majority of published articles follow a similar structure.

Title: This should be concise and informative, but sometimes an attention-grabbing title is used to attract readers to an otherwise dull paper. The title can influence the number of people who read the article, which can in turn lead to increased citations.

Author(s): This should allow you to see if the authors have the appropriate academic and professional qualifications and experience. The institutions where the authors work might also be listed and can increase the credibility of the project if they have a good reputation for research in this field. Be wary of 'guest' or 'gift' authors who did not contribute to the article. These authors might have been added to make the list of authors appear more impressive or to enhance the authors' curricula vitae. Conversely, a 'ghost' author is someone who contributed to a piece of work, but who is left uncredited despite qualifying for authorship.

Abstract: This summarises the research paper, briefly describing the reasons for doing the research, the methodology, the overall findings and the conclusions made. Reading the abstract is a quick way of getting to know the article, but the brevity of the information provided in an abstract means that it is unlikely to reveal the strengths and weaknesses of the research. If the abstract is of interest to you, you must go on to read the rest of the article. Never rely on an abstract alone to inform your medical practice!

Introduction: This explains what the research is about and why the study was carried out. A good introduction will include references to previous work related to the subject matter and describe the importance and limitations of what is already known.

Method: This section gives detailed information about how the study was actually carried out. Specific information is given on the study design, the population of interest, how the sample of the population was selected, the interventions offered and which outcomes were measured and how they were measured.

Results: This section shows what happened to the individuals studied. It might include raw data and might explain the statistical tests used to analyse the data. The results can be laid out in tables, diagrams and graphs.

Conclusion / discussion: This section discusses the results in the context of what is already known about the subject area and the clinical relevance of what has been found. It might include a discussion on the limitations of the research and suggestions on further research.

Conflicts of interests / funding: Articles should be published on their scientific merit. A conflict of interest is any factor that interferes with the objectivity of research findings. Conflicts of interest can be held by anyone involved in the research project, from the formulation of a research proposal through to its publication, including authors, their employers, a sponsoring organisation, journal editors and peer reviewers. Conflicts of interest can be financial (eg research grants, honoraria for speaking at meetings), professional (eg being a member of an organisational body) or personal (eg a relationship with the journal's editor). Ideally, authors should disclose conflicts of interest when they submit their research work. **A conflict of interest does not necessarily mean that the results of a study are void.**

Ileal-lymphoid-nodular hyperplasia, non-specific colitis, and pervasive developmental disorder in children
Wakefield AJ, Murch SH, Anthny A, et al., Lancet 1998, 351, 637–41.
This study raised the possibility of a link between the measles, mumps and rubella vaccine (MMR) given to children in their second year of life and inflammatory bowel disease and autism. This was widely reported by the media. The MMR scare reduced vaccination rates to 80% nationally, leading to a loss of herd immunity and measles outbreaks in the UK. Later it was revealed that the lead author was being funded through solicitors seeking evidence to use against vaccine manufacturers and he also had a patent for a single measles vaccine at the time of the study. Ten of the study's 13 authors later signed a formal retraction[1]. The editor of the Lancet said the research study would never have been published if he had known of a serious conflict of interest.

[1] Murch SH, Anthony A, Casson DH, et al. Retraction of an interpretation. Lancet 2004, 363, 750.

SECTION B

APPRAISING THE METHODOLOGY

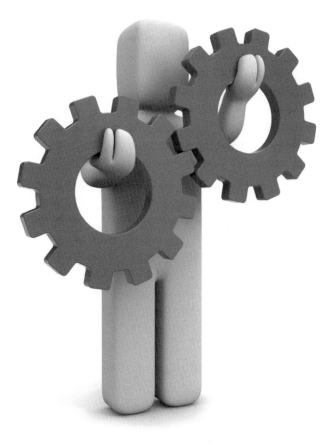

OVERVIEW OF METHODOLOGY

In a clinical paper the methodology employed to generate the results is described. Generally, the following questions need to be answered:

- What is the clinical question that needs to be answered?
- What is the study design and is it appropriate?
- How many arms are there in the study and how do they differ?
- Who are the subjects? How were they recruited and allocated to the different arms?
- What is being measured and how?
- What measures have been taken to reduce bias and confounding?
- Who funded the study and are there any competing interests?

Any shortcoming in the methodology can lead to results that do not reflect the truth. If clinical practice is changed on the basis of these results, patients could be harmed.

The researchers might highlight methodological problems in the discussion part of the paper but the onus is still on the reader to appraise the methodology carefully. Thankfully, most problems fall into two categories – bias and confounding factors. If the methodology is found to be fatally flawed, the results become meaningless and cannot be applied to clinical practice, no matter how good they are.

Researchers employ a variety of techniques to make the methodology more robust, such as matching, restriction, randomisation and blinding. In the following chapters it will become clear why these techniques are used.

Reading the methodology is therefore an active process in which strengths and weaknesses are identified.

THE CLINICAL QUESTION

Scenario 2

Dr Green, a GP, smiled as she read the final draft of her research paper. Her survey of 50 patients with fungal nail infections demonstrated that more than half of them had used a public swimming pool in the month before their infection developed. She posted a copy of the paper to her Public Health Consultant, proposing she submit the article to the Journal of Public Health.

A common misconception is that the study design is the most important determinant of the merits of a clinical paper. As soon as the words 'randomised controlled trial' appear, many clinicians assume that the study is of great value and that the results can be applied to their own clinical practice. If this approach were true, then there would be no need for any other type of study.

The critical appraisal of a paper must begin by examining the clinical question that is at the heart of the paper. **The clinical question determines which study designs are appropriate.**

- One clinical question can be answered by more than one study design.
- No single study design can answer all clinical questions.

The clinical question is normally stated in the title of the paper. The first few paragraphs of the paper should explain the reasons why the clinical question needs to be answered. There might be references to, and a discussion of, previous research and it is quite legitimate to repeat research in order to confirm earlier results.

The clinical question

There are five broad categories of clinical questions, as shown in **Table 4**.

CLINICAL QUESTION	CLINICAL RELEVANCE AND POSSIBLE STUDY DESIGNS
Aetiology/causation	What caused the disorder and how is this related to the development of the illness? Examples: case–control study, cohort study
Therapy	Which treatments do more good than harm compared with an alternative treatment? Examples: randomised control trial, systematic review, meta-analysis
Prognosis	What is the likely course of a patient's illness? What is the balance of the risks and benefits of a treatment? Examples: cohort study, longitudinal survey
Diagnosis	How valid and reliable is a diagnostic test? What does the test tell the doctor? Examples: cohort study, case–control study
Cost-effectiveness	Which intervention is worth prescribing? Is a newer treatment X worth prescribing compared with the older treatment Y? Example: economic analysis

Table 4 The different types of clinical question

The primary hypothesis

The type of clinical question determines the types of study that will be appropriate. In the methodology, the researcher must specify how the study will answer the clinical question. This will usually involve stating a hypothesis and then explaining how this hypothesis will be proved or not proved. The hypothesis is usually the same as or closely related to the clinical question. It is also known as the **a priori hypothesis** – ie the hypothesis is generated prior to data collection.

A study should, ideally, be designed and powered to answer one well-defined primary hypothesis.

If there is a secondary hypothesis, its analysis needs to be described in the same way as for the primary hypothesis. The protocol should include details of how the secondary outcomes will be analysed. Ideally, further exploratory analyses should be identified before the completion of the study and there should be a clear rationale for such analyses.

Finally, not all studies are designed to test a hypothesis. Some studies, such as case reports or qualitative studies, can be used to generate hypotheses.

Subgroup analysis

Statistical significance is discussed later in this book. Briefly, if one outcome is being measured, a statistically significant result can arise purely by chance. If two outcomes are being measured, each result can be statistically significant purely by chance, so, if the probabilities of this happening are combined, a significant result will arise more often than if only one outcome is being measured. As more outcomes are being investigated, it becomes more likely a significant result will arise by chance.

Data dredging is a problem in research studies and sometimes it can result in researchers testing for many things but only reporting the significant results. Performing many subgroup analyses has the effect of greatly increasing the chance that at least one of these comparisons will be statistically significant, even if there is no real difference (a type 1 error). For example, where several factors can influence an outcome (eg sex, age, ethnicity, smoking status) the risk of false-positive results is high. As a result, conclusions can be misleading. Deciding on subgroups after the results are available can also lead to bias.

Multiple hypothesis testing on the same set of results should therefore be avoided. Subgroup analyses should be restricted to a minimum and, if possible, subgroup analyses should be prespecified in the methodology whenever possible. Any analyses suggested by the data should be acknowledged as exploratory, for generating hypotheses and not for testing them.

In a 2010 Supplementary guidance[1] the General Medical Council states, 'Restricting research subjects to subgroups of the population that may be defined, for example, by age, gender, ethnicity or sexual orientation, for legitimate methodological reasons does not constitute discrimination.'

1   General Medical Council. *Good Practice in Research and Consent To Research* (Supplementary guidance). London, GMC, 2010.

Scenario 2 revisited

Dr Green's colleague was less enthusiastic about the findings. He wrote, 'Interesting though the results are, your chosen study design shows merely an association between swimming pools and fungal nail infections. I think you wanted to know whether a causative relationship exists. I'm afraid a cross-sectional survey cannot answer that question. Before you panic the general public, may I suggest you go back to the drawing board and, based on your question, choose a more appropriate study design?'

Self-assessment exercise 1

A study fails to meet its primary hypothesis but it is statistically significant for its secondary and tertiary hypotheses. What conclusions will you draw?

TO SUMMARISE, A GOOD STUDY WILL ...
Clearly state the clinical question or primary hypothesis
Explain why the research was done
Explain how the research differs from research already published
Specify any subgroup analyses that will be done

The type of clinical question determines the types of studies that will be appropriate.

Study designs fall into three main categories:

1. **Observational descriptive studies** – the researcher reports what has been observed in one person or in a group of people.
2. **Observational analytical studies** – the researcher reports the similarities and differences observed between two or more groups of people.
3. **Experimental studies** – the researcher intervenes in some way with one group of people and reports any differences in the outcome between this experimental group and a control group where no intervention or a different intervention was offered.

Examples of different study designs will be described in the next four chapters. The advantages and disadvantages of the different designs might include references to terms that we have not yet covered. (**Figure 5** on page 38 is a flowchart that can be used to decide on an appropriate study type.)

Terms used to describe studies

Longitudinal: Deals with a group of subjects at more than one point in time.

Cross-sectional: Deals with a group of subjects at a single point in time (ie a snapshot in time).

Prospective: Deals with the present and the future (ie looks forward).

Retrospective: Deals with the present and the past (ie looks back).

Ecological: A population or community is studied, giving information at a population level rather than at an individual level.

Pragmatic: Trials can be described as either explanatory or pragmatic. Explanatory trials tend to measure efficacy. Pragmatic trials measure effectiveness because the trials take place in ordinary clinical situations such as outpatient clinics. The results of these trials are considered to be more reflective of everyday practice, as long as the patients selected are representative of the patients who will receive the treatment. Often a new treatment is compared with a standard treatment rather than with a placebo. Pragmatic trials tend to be difficult to control and difficult to blind, and there are difficulties with excessive drop-outs.

Cluster: In these trials, people are randomly assigned to study groups as a group or cluster instead of as individuals. These trials can be useful for evaluating the delivery of health services.

OBSERVATIONAL DESCRIPTIVE STUDIES

In observational descriptive studies the researcher describes what has been observed in a sample. Nothing is done to the people in the sample. There is no control group for comparison. These studies are useful for generating ideas for research projects.

Case report

A single person is studied. Case reports are easy to write, but they tend to be anecdotal and cannot usually be repeated. They are also prone to chance association and bias. Their value lies in the fact that they can be used to generate a hypothesis.

The Medicines and Healthcare products Regulatory Agency's 'Yellow Card Scheme' is an example of case reports on patients who have suffered suspected adverse drug reactions. Yellow Card reports are evaluated each week to find previously unidentified potential hazards and other new information on the side-effects of medicines.

Case series

A group of people are studied in a case series. Case series are useful for studying rare diseases.

There are hardly any journals devoted to publishing case reports and case series alone. These studies are more likely to be found in poster presentations in conferences and as letters or rapid responses in journals. Case reports and case series are low down in the hierarchy of evidence but are useful for identifying new diseases, symptoms and signs, aetiological factors, associations, treatment approaches and prognostic factors.

A famous case series was published as a letter in the *Lancet* in 1961[1], in which WG McBride wrote, '*Sir, Congenital abnormalities are present in approximately 1.5% of babies. In recent months I have observed that the incidence of multiple severe abnormalities in babies delivered of women who were given the drug thalidomide during pregnancy, as an antiemetic or as a sedative, to be almost 20%. Have any of your readers seen similar abnormalities in babies delivered of women who have taken this drug during pregnancy?*' The link with congenital abnormalities led to the withdrawal of thalidomide from the market.

[1] McBride WG. Thalidomide and congenital abnormalities. *Lancet* 1961, 2, 1358.

OBSERVATIONAL ANALYTICAL STUDIES

In observational analytical studies the researcher reports the similarities and differences observed between subjects in two or more groups. These studies are useful for investigating the relationships between risk factors and outcomes. The two types, cohort and case–control studies, differ in their initial focus. Cohort studies focus initially on the risk factor; case–control studies focus initially on the outcome.

Cohort study

A group of subjects exposed to a risk factor are matched to a group of subjects not exposed to a risk factor. At the beginning of the study no subject has the outcome. Both groups are followed up to see how the likelihood of an outcome differs between the groups (**Figure 1**). The researcher hopes to show that subjects exposed to a risk factor are more likely to have the outcome compared with the control group.

Cohort studies are used to investigate the consequences of exposure to risk factors, so they are able to answer questions about aetiology and prognosis. They can give a direct estimation of disease incidence rates. They can also assess temporal relationships and multiple outcomes.

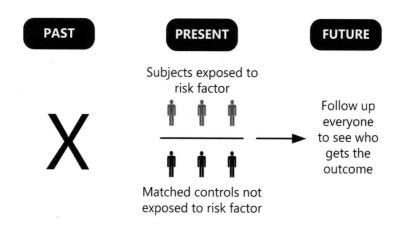

Figure 1 Cohort study design

It can take a long time from exposure to the development of the outcome. Cohort studies can be expensive to set up and maintain. Bias becomes a problem if subjects drop out of the study. Confounding factors can also be a problem. Blinding is difficult and there is no randomisation.

The mortality of doctors in relation to their smoking habits; a preliminary report
Doll R, Bradford Hill A. *British Medical Journal* 1954, 1, 1451–5.

A cohort study which examined the relationship between smoking and lung cancer: 24 389 doctors were divided into two groups, depending on whether or not they were exposed to the risk factor (smoking). Twenty-nine months later, an examination of the cause of 789 deaths revealed a significant and steadily rising mortality from deaths due to lung cancer as the amount of tobacco smoked increased.

Cohort studies are also known as 'prospective' or 'follow-up' studies.

Sometimes a study is described as a **retrospective cohort study**. This sounds paradoxical but a retrospective cohort design simply means that the researcher identified a cohort study already in progress and added another outcome of interest. This saves the researcher time and money by not having to set up another cohort from scratch.

An **inception cohort** is a group of subjects who are recruited at an early stage in the disease process but before the outcome is established.

Case–control study

Subjects who have the outcome are matched with subjects who don't have the outcome. All the subjects are asked about whether they have been exposed to one or more risk factors in the past (**Figure 2**). The researcher hopes to show that subjects with the outcome are more likely to have been exposed to the risk factor(s) compared with the control group.

Case–control studies are also known as 'case comparison' or 'retrospective' studies. They are used to investigate the causes of outcomes. They are particularly useful in situations where there is a long time period between exposure and outcome, as there is no waiting involved.

Case–control studies are usually quick and cheap to do because few subjects are required, but it can be difficult to recruit a matching control group. The major difficulty with case–control studies is the need to rely on recall and records to determine the risk factors to which the subjects have been exposed. The temporal relationship between exposure and outcome can be difficult to establish.

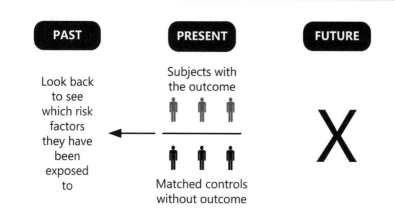

Figure 2 Case–control study design

Smoking and carcinoma of the lung: preliminary report.
Doll R, Bradford Hill A. *British Medical Journal* 1950, 2, 739–48.

A case–control study in which patients who had suspected lung, liver or bowel cancers were asked about past exposure to risk factors, including smoking. Those with lung cancer were confirmed as smokers, and those who were given the all-clear were non-smokers.

Studying rare risk factors or outcomes

If the relationship between a risk factor and disease is being investigated and the risk factor is rare, the best way to guarantee a sufficient number of people with the risk factor is by using a cohort design. It would be unwise to choose a case–control design. Case–control studies start by recruiting subjects with and subjects without an outcome. Many people would need to be recruited in order to find the few that have been exposed to the rare risk factor.

If it is the outcome that is rare, the best way to guarantee a sufficient number of people with the outcome is by using a case–control design. It would not be a good idea to choose a cohort design. Cohort studies start by recruiting subjects with and subjects without a risk factor. A large number of people would need to be followed up to detect the few who have the rare outcome.

Case–cohort and nested case–control studies

A **nested case–control study** is done in a population taking part in a cohort study. Once sufficient numbers of outcomes have been reached in the cohort population, the case–control study can be used to investigate exposures not previously taken into consideration at baseline. The cases in the study are matched to controls in the same cohort. A nested case–control study helps to reduce costs.

In a **case–cohort study** cases are recruited just as in a traditional case–control study. The difference is that the control group is recruited from everyone in the initial cohort (the population at risk at the start of the risk period), regardless of their future disease status. The control group is a sample of the full cohort.

The STROBE checklist

The 'STROBE' acronym stands for **ST**rengthening the **R**eporting of **OB**servational studies in **E**pidemiology. This is the aim of an international group of epidemiologists, methodologists, statisticians, researchers and journal editors involved in the conduct and dissemination of observational studies. Checklists for appraising cohort, case–control and cross-sectional studies can be downloaded from the STROBE website (www.strobe-statement.org).

Association or causation?

Observational analytical studies are often used to show the association between exposure to a risk factor and an outcome. Association does not necessarily imply causation, however. Deciding if a causative relationship exists is made easier by using Sir Austin Bradford Hill's nine considerations for assessing the question, 'When does association imply causation?'[1]:

- **Strength:** Is the association strong enough and large enough that we can rule out other factors?

- **Consistency:** Have the results been replicated by different researchers, in different places or circumstances and at different times?

- **Specificity:** Is the exposure associated with a very specific disease?

- **Temporality:** Did the exposure precede the disease?

- **Biological gradient:** Are increasing levels of exposure associated with an increased risk of disease?

1   Bradford Hill A. The environment and disease: association or causation? *Proceedings of the Royal Society of Medicine* 1965, 58, 295–300.

- **Plausibility:** Is there a scientific mechanism that can explain the causative relationship?
- **Coherence:** Is the association consistent with the natural history of the disease?
- **Experimental evidence:** Is there evidence from other randomised experiments?
- **Analogy:** Is any association analogous to any previously proved causal association?

For establishing whether a causal relationship exists between a microorganism and a disease, for example, **Koch's postulates**, named after the German physician, are useful, although their use is limited because there are exceptions to the rules:

- The bacteria must be present in all cases of the disease.
- The bacteria must be isolated from the host with the disease and grown in pure culture.
- The disease must be reproduced when a pure culture of the bacteria is inoculated into a healthy host.
- The bacteria must be recoverable from the experimentally infected host.

Rothman and Greenland introduced the concepts of **sufficient cause** and **component cause** to illustrate that discussing causation is rarely a straightforward matter[1]. A cause of a specific disease event was defined as an event, condition or characteristic that preceded the disease event and without which the disease event either would not have occurred at all or would not have occurred until some later time.

A 'sufficient cause', which means a complete causal mechanism, can be defined as a set of minimal conditions and events that inevitably produces disease.

It might be that no specific event, condition or characteristic is sufficient by itself to produce disease. A 'component cause' might play a role as a causal mechanism but by itself might not be a sufficient cause. The component cause must act with others to produce a causal mechanism. Component causes nearly always include some genetic and environmental factors.

Rothman's pies are used to illustrate these concepts. The pie chart is shown divided into individual component slices. The pie as a whole is the sufficient causal complex and is the combination of several component causes (the slices of the pie).

---

1   Rothman KJ, Greenland S. Causation and causal inference in epidemiology. *American Journal of Public Health* 2005, 95(Suppl 1), S144–50.

EXPERIMENTAL STUDIES

In experimental studies the researcher intervenes in some way to measure the impact of a treatment. If there is no control group, all the subjects in the study are given the same treatment.

Controlled trials

In controlled trials subjects in the study are given one of two treatments. The treatment under investigation is given to the experimental group. A standard intervention, a placebo treatment or no treatment is given to the control group for comparison. The researchers report any differences in the outcome between the experimental group and the control group.

Usually the experimental and control groups are compared together in a research project. If historical controls are used, the experimental group is compared with old data in a control group.

Some trials have more than two groups.

Randomised controlled trials

This is the gold-standard design for studying treatment effects. Subjects in the study are randomly allocated a treatment, which minimises selection bias and might equally distribute confounding factors between the treatment arms, depending on the randomisation strategy. Randomised controlled trials are a reliable measure of efficacy and allow for meta-analyses, but they are difficult, time-consuming and expensive to set up. There can be ethical problems in giving different treatments to the groups.

Crossover trials

All the subjects receive one treatment and then switch to the other treatment halfway through the study (**Figure 3**). Crossover trials are often used to study rare diseases where the lack of subjects would make a conventional trial underpowered.

The crossover design has another advantage. A researcher in a treatment study needs to ensure that the subjects in the two arms are similar, so that any difference in outcome can be attributed to the presence or absence of treatment. In a crossover study the subjects are their own controls, so matching is almost perfect. The word 'almost' is used here on purpose: usually in research studies the results in the experimental arm are compared with the results in the control arm at the same point in time (parallel arms); in a crossover design, the comparison takes place at different time points. This can be a problem if something changes that means dissimilar conditions exist at the two time points.

The researcher must also ensure that there are no carry-over effects from the first intervention that could impact on how well the subjects do with the second intervention. Carry-over effects can be caused by long half-lives and discontinuation effects. These problems can be reduced by using washout periods. The order in which the interventions are given can also be important.

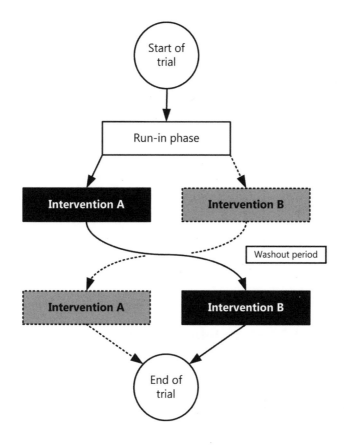

Figure 3 Crossover study design

n-of-1 trials

In an 'n-of-1' trial a single subject is studied and receives repeated courses of the active drug and alternative treatment in a random order. The subject reports on their progress regularly. This can establish effectiveness in a particular subject because it can reveal whether clinical improvement occurs only at the time of being in receipt of the active drug.

Factorial studies

Experimental trials need not limit themselves to evaluating one intervention at a time. Factorial randomised trials assess the impact of more than one intervention and can give researchers an insight into how different interventions interact with one another.

For example, a researcher might wish to randomise subjects to receive an antidepressant versus placebo and then an antipsychotic versus placebo. The different treatment groups are shown in **Table 5**.

		ANTIDEPRESSANT	
		Yes	Placebo A
ANTIPSYCHOTIC	Yes	Group 1 Antidepressant + Antipsychotic	Group 2 Placebo A + Antipsychotic
	Placebo B	Group 3 Antidepressant + Placebo B	Group 4 Placebo A + Placebo B

Table 5 Factorial trial design

The CONSORT statement

First published in the *Journal of the American Medical Association* in August 1996, the Consolidated Standards of Reporting Trials (CONSORT) statement introduced a set of recommendations to improve the quality of randomised controlled trial reports[1]. The statement was updated in 2010. This checklist is summarised in **Table 6** (further information is available at www.consort-statement.org).

1   Moher D, Schulz KF, Altman DG. The CONSORT statement: revised recommendations for improving the quality of reports of parallel-group randomised trials. *Lancet* 2001, 357, 1191–4.

SECTION OF PAPER	DESCRIPTION
Title and abstract	
	Identification as a randomised trial in the title
	Structured summary of trial design, methods, results, and conclusions (for specific guidance see CONSORT for abstracts)
Introduction	
Background and objectives	Scientific background and explanation of rationale
	Specific objectives or hypotheses
Methods	
Trial design	Description of trial design (such as parallel, factorial), including allocation ratio
	Important changes to methods after trial commencement (such as eligibility criteria), with reasons
Participants	Eligibility criteria for participants
	Settings and locations where the data were collected
Interventions	The interventions for each group with sufficient details to allow replication, including how and when they were actually administered
Outcomes	Completely defined, prespecified primary and secondary outcome measures, including how and when they were assessed
	Any changes to trial outcomes after the trial commenced, with reasons
Sample size	How sample size was determined
	When applicable, explanation of any interim analyses and stopping guidelines
Randomisation – sequence generation	Method used to generate the random allocation sequence
	Type of randomisation; details of any restriction (such as blocking and block size)

SECTION OF PAPER	DESCRIPTION
Randomisation – allocation concealment	Mechanism used to implement the random allocation sequence (such as sequentially numbered containers), describing any steps taken to conceal the sequence until interventions were assigned
Randomisation – implementation	Who generated the random allocation sequence, who enrolled participants and who assigned participants to interventions
Blinding	If done, who was blinded after assignment to interventions (eg participants, care providers, those assessing outcomes) and how If relevant, description of the similarity of interventions
Statistical methods	Statistical methods used to compare groups for primary and secondary outcomes Methods for additional analyses, such as subgroup analyses and adjusted analyses
Results	
Participant flow	For each group, the numbers of participants who were randomly assigned, received intended treatment and were analysed for the primary outcome For each group, losses and exclusions after randomisation, together with reasons
Recruitment	Dates defining the periods of recruitment and follow-up Why the trial ended or was stopped
Baseline data	A table showing baseline demographic and clinical characteristics for each group
Numbers analysed	For each group, number of participants (denominator) included in each analysis and whether the analysis was by original assigned groups
Outcomes and estimation	For each primary and secondary outcome, results for each group and the estimated effect size and its precision (such as 95% confidence interval) For binary outcomes, presentation of both absolute and relative effect sizes is recommended

SECTION OF PAPER	DESCRIPTION
Ancillary analyses	Results of any other analyses performed, including subgroup analyses and adjusted analyses, distinguishing prespecified from exploratory
Harms	All important harms or unintended effects in each group
Discussion	
Limitations	Trial limitations, addressing sources of potential bias, imprecision and, if relevant, multiplicity of analyses
Generalisability	Generalisability (external validity, applicability) of the trial findings
Interpretation	Interpretation consistent with results, balancing benefits and harms and considering other relevant evidence
Other information	
Registration	Registration number and name of trial registry
Protocol	Where the full trial protocol can be accessed, if available
Funding	Sources of funding and other support (such as supply of drugs), role of funders

The Standards for Quality Improvement Reporting Excellence (SQUIRE) Group have also published guidelines to improve standards[1] (guidelines available at www.squire-statement.org).

1   Davidoff F, Batalden P, Stevens D, Ogrine G, Mooney SE. Publication guidelines for quality improvement studies in health care: evolution of the SQUIRE project. BMJ 2009, 338, a3152.

Audit

Aspects of service provision are assessed against a gold standard, which can be a national guideline, a local protocol or generally accepted best practice. Sometimes it is necessary to devise a gold standard in the absence of a published one.

Data on the service are collected and compared with the gold standard. A change is then implemented in the running of the service and the audit cycle is completed by another collection of data (**Figure 4**).

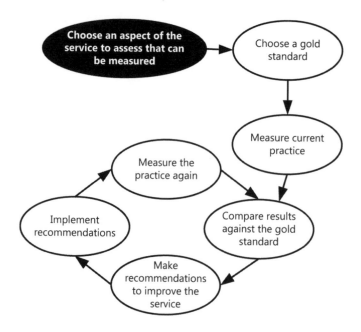

Figure 4 The audit cycle

Audits provide information on the effectiveness of services, but they are resource-hungry and take clinicians away from clinical work. Audits do not usually require ethical approval.

Surveys

In a survey a group of subjects is questioned. Surveys can identify patterns and help to plan service provision. Surveys cannot distinguish between cause and effect.

In a **qualitative survey** opinions are elicited from a group of subjects, with the emphasis on the subjective meaning and experience. Such studies can be used to study complex issues. The inquiry can be via interviews, focus groups or participant observation. However, it can be difficult to get information, record it and analyse the subjective data.

In a **cross-sectional survey**, subjects are questioned for the presence of risk factors and outcomes. They are useful for establishing prevalence. They establish association, not causality. Such surveys are cheap and simple and are ethically safe. The groups can be unequal, confounders can be asymmetrically distributed and recall bias is a problem. Large numbers of subjects are usually required.

Surveys are usually used to collect information on a sample of the population. A **census** is a special kind of survey in which data on every person and/or household in a population are collected.

Economic analysis

This type of study assesses the cost and/or utilities of intervention. Such analyses help to prioritise services, but it is difficult to remain objective because assumptions have to be made.

Systematic review and meta-analysis

A systematic review attempts to access and review systematically all of the pertinent articles in the field. A meta-analysis combines the results of several studies and produces a quantitative assessment.

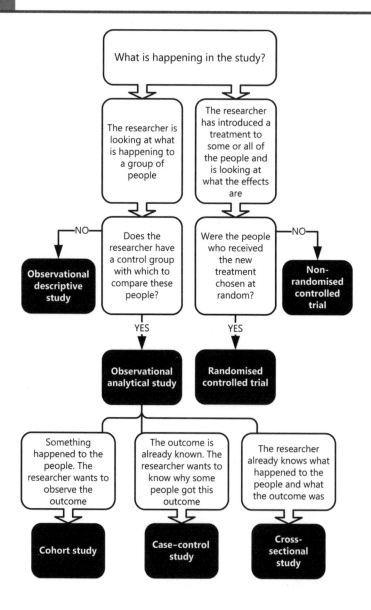

Figure 5 Distinguishing between study types

Self-assessment exercise 2

What types of studies are suggested by the following statements?

1. Patients with ankle injuries who are seeing a physiotherapist are questioned about the type of trainers they wear in order to investigate the relationship between running shoes and susceptibility to ankle injuries. There answers are compared with those of healthy people.

2. Builders exposed to asbestos on a demolition site are seen regularly, to detect any adverse consequences.

3. A consultant physician investigates how many patients newly referred to the outpatient clinic are seen within 16 weeks of the date of referral.

4. Patients with chronic lower back pain are randomly given one of two treatments and assessed regularly.

5. Residents in a leafy suburb are questioned about their opinions on whether planning permission should be given for a new psychiatric medium-secure unit in the neighbourhood.

6. The commissioners investigate whether to reallocate funds originally set aside for an obesity clinic to a new treatment for bowel cancer instead.

Self-assessment exercise 3

1. You have developed a blood test for detecting meningitis. How will you set up a study to see if your test is any good?

2. You have developed a new treatment for patients with anorexia nervosa. How will you set up a study to see if your new treatment is any good?

3. You suspect that smoking cannabis leads to the onset of schizophrenia. How will you set up a study to see if this is true?

4. You think that outpatients who are diagnosed with a frozen shoulder will never return to work. How will you set up a study to see if your suspicions are right?

Self-assessment exercise 4

1. What are the advantages and disadvantages of a crossover design compared with a traditional randomised controlled trial?

2. How do cohort studies differ from case–control studies? Which is preferred for investigating the effect of rare exposures? Which is preferred for investigating the cause of rare outcomes?

3. What restriction is imposed on the choice of topics that you as a clinician can audit?

Bringing a drug to the market can take several years and cost hundreds of millions of pounds (**Figure 6**). The developmental process usually begins with the identification of a biological target that is linked with the aetiology of a disease. Compounds are formulated to act on this target. The chosen compound is then transformed and packaged in such a way that it can be administered to patients to give the maximum benefit and the minimum of side-effects. This transformation process involves a series of trials on animals and humans that are subject to the rigorous controls required by the regulatory authorities and local ethics committees.

Clinical trial authorisations are needed for all new products in development. Applications for such authorisations in the UK are assessed by the medical, pharmaceutical and scientific staff at the Medicines and Healthcare products Regulatory Agency (MHRA), an agency of the Department of Health.

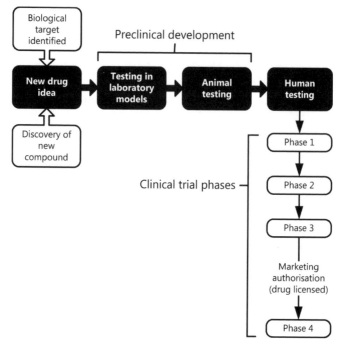

Figure 6 The research pathway

Clinical trial phases

Clinical trials of experimental drugs consist of four phases.

Phase 1 clinical trials

These are the earliest trials in the life of a new drug or treatment. The researchers test a new drug or treatment in a small group of **healthy people** for the first time, to assess its safety, establish a dosage range and identify any side-effects. These trials aim to help in the evaluation and understanding of the behaviour of the molecule or compound. The healthy volunteers are normally compensated for the time they are giving up but are not given financial incentives to take part in research.

Phase 2 clinical trials

About seven out of every ten new treatments tested at phase 1 in healthy volunteers proceed to phase 2 trials and are tested on **people with the relevant illness**. At this stage, the study drug or treatment is given to a larger group of people to assess its effectiveness and safety profile.

Phase 3 clinical trials

At this stage, the study drug or treatment is given to large groups of **people in clinical settings** to make further assessments of its effectiveness, dose range and duration of treatment, and to monitor side-effects. These trials compare the new treatment with the best currently available treatment (the standard treatment).

Providing satisfactory results are gained from phase 3 studies, a drug will get a **marketing authorisation**, which sets out its agreed terms and conditions of use, such as indications and dosage. Even drugs with a high risk-to-benefit ratio can be approved, for example if the drug enhances the quality of life of patients with terminal illnesses.

Phase 4 clinical trials

Phase 4 trials, also known as **post-marketing surveillance studies**, are carried out after a drug has been shown to work, has been granted a licence and been marketed. Information is collected about the benefits and side-effects of the drug in different populations. Data on long-term usage are also collected. These studies involve monitoring the safety of medicines under their usual conditions of use, and they can also be carried out to identify any new safety concerns (**hypothesis generating**) and to confirm or refute these concerns (**hypothesis testing**).

POPULATIONS AND SAMPLES

Researchers identify the target population they are interested in. It is rarely feasible to include everyone in the target population in the trial. A sample population is therefore taken and results from this sample are then generalised to the target population (**Figure 7**). The size of the sample population can be determined by a power calculation.

The sample should be representative of the target population from which it came. Knowing the **baseline characteristics** of the sample population is important because this allows doctors to see how closely the subjects match their own patients. Such characteristics can include demographic characteristics, such as age and sex, as well as more fluid variables, such as smoking status. These details are often displayed in the form of a table in the research paper.

When we consider the applicability of research findings, we are usually asking firstly whether the sample population in the study is representative of the target population and, secondly, whether our patients match those in the study's target population. If the sample population is unrepresentative or the target population is unlike our own, the research findings might not be applicable to our patients, no matter how good the evidence.

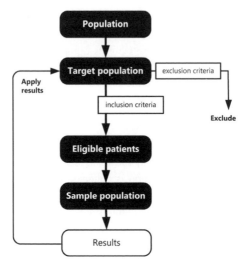

Figure 7 How the people at different stages of a study are described

Methods of sampling

There are five common techniques that are used to obtain a sample from a population:

1. **(Simple) random sampling:** Every person in the target population has an equal chance of being selected. Random sampling is also known as **representative sampling** or **proportionate sampling** because all groups should be proportionately represented.

2. **Systematic sampling:** Every nth member of the target population is selected once the first person has been chosen at random. This is also known as **quasi-random sampling**. It usually gives a representative sample of the population.

3. **Stratified sampling:** Different populations of people are recruited from particular subgroups or strata in the target population. This is achieved by dividing the target population into two or more strata based on one or more characteristics, and sampling each stratum (usually randomly).

4. **Cluster sampling:** The target population is divided into clusters and some of these clusters are exhaustively sampled.

5. **Convenience sampling:** Sampling is done as convenient, often allowing the subject to choose whether or not he or she is sampled. Convenience sampling is the easiest and potentially most dangerous. Good results can often be obtained, but just as often the data set can be seriously **biased**.

TO SUMMARISE, A GOOD STUDY WILL ...

Describe the target population

Explain how the sample population was recruited

Explain how the sample size was determined

Comment on how well the sample population represents the target population

BIAS

Scenario 3

Mr Pahal, Consultant Plastic Surgeon, was interested in how many patients would use a hospital website to access information about postoperative care. He placed an advertisement in The Times newspaper and recruited 90 people for his survey. He concluded that 70% of patients would definitely visit a hospital website for more information about the management of surgical wounds. He put forward a proposal to the Hospital Board for funding the development of such a website.

Scenario 4

Consultant Psychiatrist, Dr Thomas, had a long-standing interest in the treatment of anxiety disorders. Her Clinical Director wanted her to set up a specialist clinic for patients with anxiety disorders, but needed to justify the expense to the Hospital Board. Dr Thomas sent a postal questionnaire to 500 patients of the Psychiatry Unit, asking them if they had ever been told they had a neurotic disorder. If the answer was 'yes', she asked them to describe the treatments offered and whether they would support the development of a specialist clinic.

Scenario 5

Nurse Smith wanted to illustrate the quality of care provided by her team to patients on a gastroenterology ward. She visited every patient on the day of their discharge home and took them through a questionnaire to rate the quality of the care they received during their hospital stay. She presented the near-perfect results to the matron and asked for a salary increase.

Errors in studies can lead to results that are misleading and conclusions that are wrong. For example, interventions and treatments might appear more or less beneficial than they actually are. Errors in studies can happen either by chance or through mistakes in the way the study was done.

Bias is the term used to describe an error at any stage of the study that was not due to chance. Bias undermines the internal validity of the study and impacts on the external validity of findings. Bias leads to results in which there is a systematic deviation from the truth. As bias cannot be measured or controlled for statistically, researchers need to rely on good research design to minimise bias.

There are many types of bias and many ways of classifying them. The main types of bias can be listed either at the stage of the study at which they arise or in the broad categories of reporting, selection, performance, observation and attrition bias (**Table 7**).

STAGE OF STUDY	CATEGORIES OF BIAS	EXAMPLES OF BIAS	EXAMPLES OF AVOIDING BIAS
Literature review	Reporting	Literature search bias	Comprehensive search strategy
		Foreign language exclusion bias	Translation
Recruitment of a sample population	Selection	Sampling bias (researcher): – Berkson bias – Diagnostic purity bias – Neyman bias – Membership bias – Historical control bias	Randomisation Concealed allocation
		Response bias (subjects)	
Running the trial	Performance	Instrument bias Questionnaire bias	Blinding
Collecting information	Observation	Interviewer bias Recall bias Response bias Hawthorne effect	Blinding outcome assessment
Analysing the results	Attrition	Attrition (exclusion) bias	Intention-to-treat analysis

Table 7 The different types of bias

Selection bias

This occurs through the identification and/or recruitment of an unrepresentative sample population. The sample population differs in some significant way from the population that generated the sample population, such that any results and conclusions drawn from the sample population cannot be generalised to the population as a whole.

Selection bias can be further divided into sampling bias, which is introduced by the researchers, and response bias, which is introduced by the study population.

Examples of **sampling bias** include:

- **Berkson (admission rate) bias:** This arises when the sample population is taken from a hospital setting, but the hospital cases do not reflect the rate or severity of the condition in the population. The relationship between exposure and disease is unrepresentative of the real situation.

- **Diagnostic purity bias:** This arises when comorbidity is excluded in the sample population, such that the sample population does not reflect the true complexity of cases in the population.

- **Neyman (incidence / prevalence) bias:** This occurs when the prevalence of a condition does not reflect its incidence. Usually this is due to a time gap between the onset of a condition and the actual selection of the study population, such that some individuals with the condition are not available for selection.

- **Membership bias:** This arises when membership of a group is used to identify study individuals. The members of such a group might not be representative of the population.

- **Historical control bias:** This arises when subjects and controls are chosen across time, such that secular changes in definitions, exposures, diseases and treatments can mean that such subjects and controls cannot be compared with one another.

Response bias occurs when individuals volunteer for studies but they differ in some way from the population. The most common reason for such a difference is that the volunteers are more motivated to improve their health and therefore participate more readily and adhere to the trial conditions better. Confusingly, the term 'response bias' can also be used to describe an observation bias (see page 47).

Even if steps are taken to reduce the risk of selection bias, a **sampling error** can also happen by chance. Large sample sizes and probability sampling help to minimise sampling error.

Selection bias can happen not only at the recruitment stage of a study but also when subjects are allocated to different arms. The group of subjects in each arm should be representative of the target population. If the subjects are not representative, a selection bias has occurred during the allocation process.

Performance bias

Performance bias occurs when differences arise in the care that is provided to the subjects in the different arms or in different centres in multicentre trials.

Observation bias

Observation bias, also known as 'information bias', occurs as a result of failure to measure or classify the exposure or outcomes correctly. It can be due to the researchers or the subjects.

Examples of observation bias include:

- **Interviewer (ascertainment) bias:** This arises when the researcher is not blinded to the subject's status in the study and this alters the researcher's approach to the subject and the recording of results.
- **Recall bias:** This arises when subjects selectively remember details from the past. This can be particularly important in case–control studies and in cross-sectional surveys.
- **Response bias:** This arises in any study in which the subjects answer questions in the way they believe the researcher wants them to answer, rather than according to their true beliefs.
- **Hawthorne effect:** This arises when subjects alter their behaviour, usually positively, because they are aware they are being observed in a study.

Attrition bias

Attrition bias arises when the numbers of individuals dropping out of the study differ significantly in the different arms of the study. Those left at the end of the study might not be representative of the study sample that was randomised at the start.

Scenario 3 revisited

Mr Pahal's proposal was rejected by the Hospital Board. In their conclusions, they commented, 'A non-representative sample was used to generate the findings. The population that the hospital serves is dissimilar to that which reads The Times *newspaper in a number of respects, including, but not limited to, lower literacy levels and less internet access. Mr Pahal should consider selecting a more representative sample for future proposals, to avoid selection bias.'*

Scenario 4 revisited

Dr Thomas's survey generated a surprising result, with only 1% of the sample having been diagnosed with a neurotic disorder. Her Clinical Director wrote to her, stating, 'Perhaps nowadays not many people are familiar with the term "neurotic". The use of the word "anxiety" might produce different results as it will eliminate observation bias. Please repeat the survey.'

Scenario 5 revisited

The matron was less than impressed. She commented, 'The results are good but what else did you expect if you asked patients about their views? They're hardly likely to give you negative comments. Perhaps I should ask an independent organisation to survey the patients at home? That will eliminate a response bias. I'm afraid a salary rise cannot be justified at this time. Now, back to work!'

Self-assessment exercise 5

For each of the following study protocols, decide if selection and/or observation bias could occur:

1. **Study aim:** To plan the provision of stroke services for elderly patients.
   Proposed method: A cross-sectional survey to discover the prevalence of cerebrovascular accidents by phoning 5000 residents across the city.

2. **Study aim:** To elicit the magnitude of drug problems in the teenage population.
   Proposed method: A survey of teenagers in all the schools in the city, asking them about illicit use of drugs.

3. **Study aim:** To investigate the association between smoking and lung cancer.
   Proposed method: A case–control study of inpatients in a respiratory disease ward in a district general hospital.

4. **Study aim:** To establish the effectiveness of pain relief offered to women during childbirth.
   Proposed method: A questionnaire sent to new mothers asking them about their experience of pain during delivery.

TO SUMMARISE, A GOOD STUDY WILL ...

Explain how the selection process minimised selection bias

Explain what techniques were employed to minimise observation bias

Acknowledge any mistakes or methodological compromises that were made

Make suggestions on how any mistakes can be avoided in future research, if possible

Scenario 6

Dr Edwards designed a case–control study to investigate the relationship between alcohol consumption and lung cancer. She recruited 700 people into her study, both healthy controls and people with lung cancer. She questioned each person on their alcohol history. To her surprise, she found a significant relationship, showing that alcohol consumption increased the risk of lung cancer, such that the finding was unlikely to have happened by chance alone. She submitted her article to the British Medical Journal.

Many studies look at the relationship between an exposure and an outcome, hoping to show that a causal relationship exists. The findings can, however, be explained by the existence of a third factor, a confounder.

A confounder has a triangular relationship with both the exposure and the outcome, but, most importantly, it is not on the causal pathway (**Figure 8**). It makes it appear as if there is a direct relationship between the exposure and the outcome or it might even mask an association that would otherwise have been present.

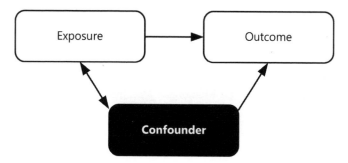

Figure 8 The relationship between the exposure, the outcome and the confounder

To be a confounding factor, the variable must be associated with:

- The exposure, but must not be the consequence of the exposure
- The outcome, independently of the exposure (ie not an intermediary)

In the example in **Figure 9**, drinking coffee appears to cause coronary heart disease. Smoking is a confounding factor. It is associated with coffee drinking and it is a risk factor for coronary heart disease, even in people who do not drink coffee.

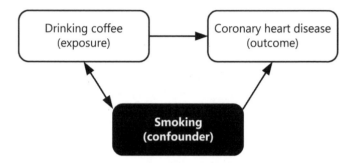

Figure 9 Smoking is a confounding factor

The reverse is not true. Coffee drinking does not confound the relationship between smoking and coronary heart disease, even though it is associated with smoking. Drinking coffee is not a risk factor for coronary heart disease independently of smoking (**Figure 10**).

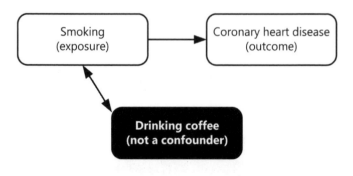

Figure 10 Drinking coffee is not a confounding factor

A **positive confounder** results in an association between two variables that are not associated:

- Example: The association between coffee drinking and lung cancer is positively confounded by smoking. People who drink coffee might also smoke. Smoking is a risk factor for lung cancer, even for those people who do not drink coffee.

A **negative confounder** masks an association that is really present:

- Example: The association between poor diet and coronary heart disease can be negatively confounded by exercise. People who exercise regularly might compensate for the effects of a poor diet, making it appear that poor diet is not associated with coronary heart disease.

Confounding can cause overestimation or underestimation of the true association and can even change the direction of the observed effect. An example is the confounding by age of an inverse association between level of exercise and heart attacks (younger people taking more rigorous exercise), causing overestimation.

Identification of confounders

Confounding factors differ from bias in that confounding is not usually created by some mistake made by the researchers. Confounding usually arises from a real-life relationship that already exists between the exposures being examined and the outcomes under consideration.

Importantly, confounding factors must be identified so that measures can be taken to eliminate them, spread them equally between different arms of the study or neutralise their effects on the results, using statistical techniques.

Confounders can be measured and controlled for (eg by multiple linear regression) but good study design is essential because you cannot exclude a confounder that was not measured.

Methods to control confounding
At the time of designing the study

- **Restriction:** Certain confounding factors are restricted from entering the sample population using inclusion and exclusion criteria.
- **Matching:** People with confounding factors are allocated equally in the different arms of a study.
- **Randomisation:** Confounding factors, known or unknown, can be evenly distributed among the study groups, depending on the method of randomisation.

Confounders can exert effects only if they differ between study groups. Restriction or matching can limit the sample size and possible analysis strategies; in particular, one cannot study the effect of a matched variable on an outcome.

At the time of analysis of the study

- Stratification
- Standardisation
- Statistical adjustment

Stratification

If a potential confounding factor can be identified in the design stage, the data generated during the study can be separated into strata on the basis of that potential confounding factor. This enables the researcher to keep the characteristics of the participants as similar as possible across the study groups (eg with regard to age, weight or functional status). Once these strata are identified, separate block randomisation schemes are created for each factor, to ensure that the groups are balanced within each stratum.

Stratification can be achieved by a statistical technique called the Mantel–Haenszel method, which gives adjusted relative risks as a summary measure of the overall risk, or as the Mantel–Haenszel estimate of odds ratio, which gives a weighted average of the strata-specific odds ratios, the weights being dependent on the numbers of observations in each stratum.

Stratification is not able to control simultaneously for even a moderate number of potential confounders. The number of strata is limited by the sample size needed for each stratum.

Standardisation

The risk in the exposed group is adjusted to that which would have been observed had there been the same confounder distribution as in the unexposed group. For example, if age is a confounding factor, the risk in the exposed group could be adjusted to the age-standardised risk. Standardisation is flexible and reversible. Data collection can be completed before potential confounders are dealt with. However, standardisation becomes difficult when dealing with more than one confounder.

Statistical adjustment using multivariate statistics

This statistical method is used to take confounding factors into account. It analyses the data by using a mathematical model that takes the outcome under consideration as the dependent variable and includes the causal factor and any confounding factors in the equation. These factors are referred to as 'covariables'. The equation allows you to check how much the confounding factors / covariables contribute to the overall effect. When the dependent variables are continuous in nature, multiple linear regression is used. If the variables are binary, logistic regression is used. The advantage of using multivariate analysis is that more than one potential confounder can be considered and the technique is flexible and reversible.

Multivariate statistics can control for a number of confounding factors simultaneously as long as there are at least 10 subjects for every variable investigated in a logistic regression situation.

Scenario 6 revisited

Dr Edwards received a letter from the editor of the British Medical Journal. The editor wrote, 'Although a most interesting conclusion, the results of the study are less impressive when confounding variables are considered. Unfortunately, smoking as a confounder has been overlooked. I'm afraid that we cannot consider publishing your study results. I wish you better luck in the future.'

Self-assessment exercise 6

In the following lists of three variables, state which factor, if not identified, would act as a confounding factor in the relationship between the other two variables:

1. Cigarette lighter, smoking cigarettes, lung cancer

2. Skin cancer, fair skin, blue eyes

3. Smoking, the oral contraceptive pill, myocardial infarction

4. Life events, poverty, depression

TO SUMMARISE, A GOOD STUDY WILL ...

List confounding factors and explain their impact on any relationship under investigation

Describe how confounding factors were controlled at the design and analysis stages

RESTRICTION

Inclusion criteria and exclusion criteria should normally be listed in the methodology section of a clinical paper.

Inclusion criteria

These criteria determine which people in the target population are eligible to be included in the sample population of a study.

Exclusion criteria

These criteria determine which people in the target population are not eligible to be included in the sample population of a study. Exclusion criteria might include ethical considerations. They can be used to eliminate known confounding factors from a study.

In order to minimise selection bias, the inclusion and exclusion criteria must be clearly stated before the study begins. Excessive use of inclusion and exclusion criteria should be avoided. Not only will it make it harder to recruit a sample population, it will also influence the generalisability of the results, as over-restriction of the sample population will make it unrepresentative of the target population (diagnostic purity bias).

Self-assessment exercise 7

You are developing a study protocol looking at the benefits of the antipsychotic drug risperidone in the treatment of schizoaffective disorder in hospital inpatients. Which inclusion and exclusion criteria would you apply?

TO SUMMARISE, A GOOD STUDY WILL ...

List the inclusion criteria and relate them to the aims of the study

List the exclusion criteria and explain the role of confounding factors in any relationship under investigation

Illustrate how many people were included and excluded, often in the form of a table or flowchart

Ideally, in a study with more than one arm the subjects in each arm should be as similar as possible apart from exposure to the risk factor or intervention of interest.

In case–control and cohort studies, the researchers recruit the cases first before recruiting a control group. The cases and controls are usually matched, which means that for every case there is a control subject who has similar values of the matching variables. The matching variables are usually demographic characteristics such as sex, gender and ethnicity. The variables are not of interest in themselves.

Matching can also be used to distribute confounding factors evenly. Study participants are chosen to ensure that potential confounding variables are evenly distributed in the two groups being compared. This ensures that any confounding factor that has been identified in the experimental group can also be replicated in the control group.

Matching must be used with caution because, like restriction, it can limit the sample size and possible analysis strategies. It can be difficult to find matching controls, especially with large numbers of matching variables. In these situations, matching may be abandoned in favour of using statistical analyses later on to adjust for those variables which would have been matched had there been a sufficient number of controls. This is easier to do in large studies. In small studies, matching is preferred.

There might be a table in a clinical paper comparing the baseline characteristics of subjects in the different arms. A failure of matching is shown by a significant difference in one or more characteristics between the arms.

TO SUMMARISE, A GOOD STUDY WILL ...

Describe potential confounding factors

Describe how matching was done and any difficulties encountered

Provide a table comparing the baseline demographic and prognostic characteristics of the different groups

RANDOMISATION

This method ensures that all the people entering into a study have an equal chance of being allocated to any group within the study. Allocation of subjects to specific treatment groups in a random fashion ensures that each group is, on average, as similar as possible to the other group(s).

Randomisation can be divided into three broad areas that all overlap:

- Random number generation
- Randomisation method
- Concealed allocation

Note that random sampling is not the same as randomisation. Random sampling is used to recruit a sample population from the target population. Randomisation aims to allocate subjects in the sample population to one of the intervention groups.

Random number generation

Successful randomisation requires that group assignment cannot be predicted in advance. Some methods of allocation, such as alternate allocation to treatment group or methods based on patient characteristics, are not reliably random. These allocation sequences are predictable and not easily concealed and can therefore reduce the guarantee that allocation has been random and that no potential participants have been excluded by pre-existing knowledge of the intervention.

Instead, researchers use a variety of techniques to generate a random sequence that can be used to decide allocation:

- Computer random number generation – the most popular method
- Random number tables – contain a series of numbers that occur equally often and which are arranged in a random fashion; numbers usually have two or more digits
- Shuffled cards or envelopes

Randomisation methods

Randomisation methods can be divided into:

- **Fixed randomisation:** The randomisation methods are defined and allocation sequences are set up before the start of the trial. Examples include simple randomisation, block randomisation, stratified randomisation and randomised consent.

- **Adaptive randomisation:** The randomised groups are adjusted as the study progresses to account for imbalances in the numbers in the groups or in response to the outcome data. An example is minimisation.

Fixed randomisation

Simple randomisation

Each subject's allocation is decided at random as each subject is recruited into the study, independently of any other factors. Methods include flipping a coin (for studies with two groups), rolling a die (for studies with two or more groups), random number tables and computer-generated random numbers.

With simple randomisation, confounding factors, known and unknown, have an equal chance of entering either group but at any one time the result can still be unequal group sizes and unequal distribution of confounding factors, particularly in small trials.

Block randomisation

Block randomisation is used to ensure that there are equal numbers of patients in each arm. When subjects are recruited into the sample population, they are not allocated immediately as individuals in the same way as they are in simple randomisation. Instead, subjects are put into blocks which, when filled, are divided equally into the different arms of the study. The order of this allocation within the block is randomly permuted. Some clinical papers refer to this method as 'permuted block randomisation'.

Stratified randomisation

Simple and block randomisation might not distribute confounding factors equally into the groups. Although the asymmetrical distribution of confounding factors can be dealt with using statistical analyses later on, an extension of block randomisation – stratified randomisation – can also help.

In stratified randomisation, subgroups (or strata) containing confounding factors are formed. Block randomisation takes place within each subgroup. As a result, the confounding factor is equally distributed in the different arms.

In small studies it becomes impractical to stratify on more than one or two confounding factors. Minimisation is an alternative method for achieving similarity between study arms.

Other forms of randomisation:

Randomised consent method: This is a method used when the study is interested in the effects of informed consent on treatment efficacy and on the efficacies of the compared treatments.

Quasi-random allocation: A method of allocating subjects to different arms that is not truly random. For example, subjects could be allocated by date of birth, day of the week, medical record number, month of the year or the order in which they were included in the study (alternation). A quasi-randomised trial uses a quasi-random method of allocating participants to different interventions. There is a greater risk of selection bias in quasi-random trials where allocation is not adequately concealed compared with randomised controlled trials with adequate allocation concealment.

Cluster randomisation: Subjects are not randomised as individuals. Instead, a group of subjects, or a cluster, is randomised to the same arm together. In these studies the unit of analysis is the cluster, rather than the individual subjects in that arm. A summary statistic for the improvement in each cluster is often calculated and compared. Cluster randomisation is most commonly seen in public-health and primary-care research. Cluster randomisation is not without problems. Firstly, clusters might be of different sizes yet be given equal weighting in the analysis. Secondly, as fewer data are generated by analysing clusters than would be generated by analysing individuals, the study loses power. Thirdly, individuals within a cluster tend to be more similar to each other than to members of other clusters, which can lead to an overestimation of the difference between the arms that has been caused by the intervention under investigation.

Adaptive randomisation

In adaptive randomisation methods the probability of being allocated to a certain arm in the study is adjusted to maintain similarity between the arms. As an arm becomes imbalanced with subjects of a certain characteristic, the probability of future similar subjects also being allocated to the same arm reduces.

Minimisation is the most commonly used adaptive randomisation method. At the outset the researchers decide which factors they would like to be present in equal numbers in the different arms. The first subject recruited is allocated to an arm by a random method. Following subjects are allocated to the arm in such a way as to keep all the arms as similar as possible with regard to the predetermined factors. The allocation of each subject therefore depends on the characteristics of the subjects already enrolled. In small studies minimisation is more effective than randomisation in ensuring that the different arms are as similar as possible. Minimisation is also effective when multiple factors need to be distributed evenly.

TO SUMMARISE, A GOOD STUDY WILL ...

Describe how random numbers were generated and by whom

Describe the randomisation method that was employed

Provide a table comparing the baseline demographic and prognostic characteristics of the different groups to show randomisation was effective

Discuss how concealed allocation was achieved and monitored

Scenario 7

Dr Robertson assessed an elderly woman with breathing difficulties and decided that she needed hospital treatment. He admitted the woman to a respiratory ward. The ward nurse asked if the patient was eligible for the study he was doing on the efficacy of a new nebuliser treatment. Dr Robertson replied that as the next subject to be recruited was to be allocated to the new treatment arm, he did not think he could risk it with this poorly patient, even though she met the inclusion criteria. He told the ward nurse that the patient would not be taking part in the trial.

The recruitment of subjects into a trial can be adversely affected if the interventions that will be given in each group are known. For example, the ideal result in a treatment study is a significant difference in the outcomes of subjects in the treatment and placebo groups in favour of the new treatment. This difference can be exaggerated by recruiting the 'best' patients to the treatment group and the 'worst' patients to the placebo group.

This problem can arise even if randomisation is used to allocate patients to groups because the randomisation schedule is often published in advance. If it is known that the next individual will be allocated to the new treatment group according to the randomisation schedule, an individual who is not expected to do well might be overlooked for recruitment into the study. Instead, the researcher might wait for someone who will do very well in the new treatment group. A selection bias will result as the subjects in each group are not representative of the target population.

Concealed allocation

Concealment means the interventions in the different arms of the study are kept secret. As a result, the researchers are unaware of the intervention in the group to which a subject will be allocated, should that individual agree to be in the study. This avoids both conscious and subconscious selection of patients into the study. Concealed allocation is a vital part of the randomisation process and protects against selection bias.

A good study will not have the same people recruiting and randomising subjects.

There are a number of ways in which concealed allocation can be achieved. For example, with a centralised concealment scheme in a multicentre trial, the clinician checks for eligibility, gains consent, decides on whether to enrol patients and then contacts the randomisation service to obtain the treatment allocation. This contact can be made by telephone or electronically on the internet.

In situations in which remote randomisation might not be feasible, a set of tamper-evident envelopes that look identical may be provided to each site. The envelopes are opaque and sealed, and the sequence of opening the envelopes is monitored regularly. Another technique is to use coded containers in which treatments from numbered bottles that appear otherwise identical are administered sequentially.

Concealed allocation and blinding

These two terms are often confused because they both involve keeping interventions secret. Concealed allocation is part of the randomisation and allocation procedures. It seeks to eliminate selection bias. Blinding happens after randomisation and aims to reduce observation bias (see pages 65–67).

Scenario 7 revisited

Dr Robertson's study concluded that the new nebuliser treatment was of major benefit to patients with breathing difficulties and it would save lives if it was given as a first-line treatment. He presented his findings at the hospital's academic meeting and received a standing ovation. The ward nurse was in the audience. At the end of the presentation, when Dr Robertson invited questions and comments, she said, 'As you were aware of the treatments being given in each group and the allocation sequence, your selection of patients was biased and ended up widening the difference between the groups. Does selection bias not make your results invalid?'

TO SUMMARISE, A GOOD STUDY WILL ...
Include concealed allocation as part of the randomisation process
Describe the people involved in recruiting and allocating subjects
Discuss how concealed allocation was achieved and monitored

THE PLACEBO EFFECT

Scenario 8

Dr Singh, a rheumatologist, finished writing her first case report. She had seen a patient with arthritis. The patient had visited his GP and had, by the press of a wrong key on the computer, been mistakenly dispensed co-careldopa, a treatment for Parkinson's disease, instead of co-codamol, a painkiller. The patient had unwittingly taken the wrong treatment for a month and, far from experiencing no effect, his pain symptoms had dramatically improved. Dr Singh submitted her report to the Lancet, stating that this case had demonstrated for the first time the painkilling properties of anti-parkinsonism treatment and could lead to a new treatment approach.

Researchers in intervention trials attempt to show whether a treatment improves the health of the subjects. However, subjects can improve simply if they expect to get better with treatment. This effect is so powerful that subjects can improve even if they are unaware that they have been given a placebo, or dummy treatment. A placebo does not have any therapeutic activity for the condition being treated.

Placebo effect

The placebo effect is the name given to the improvement seen in subjects when they are in receipt of a placebo treatment. The placebo effect is greater when a subject is given several pills instead of one pill, larger pills instead of smaller pills, and capsules instead of tablets.

One arm in an intervention trial is usually given the active treatment and the other arm is given a placebo treatment. The placebo is used to determine whether any difference in outcome is attributable to the active treatment or to the effect of expectation. If the improvement in the active arm is the same as that in the placebo arm, all the improvement can be attributed to the placebo effect. If the improvement is greater in the active arm, the active treatment is having a beneficial effect over and above that due to the placebo effect.

Placebos

People do not enter clinical trials hoping to be allocated to the placebo arm. However, most trials need subjects in the placebo arm. Placebo treatments should be as similar as possible to the active treatment. They should look the same, feel the same, smell the same, taste the same and have the same mode of delivery. A placebo treatment can be sourced from the manufacturer of the active treatment in order to look as similar as possible and only differ in that it has no therapeutic activity. Subjects will then be unable to determine whether they are in the placebo arm and are more likely to continue in the trial.

Some organisations argue that all new treatments should be compared in head-to-head trials with the current standard or best treatment, to see if the new treatment is significantly better. However, trials in which an active treatment is not compared with a placebo treatment cannot determine how much of any improvement is due to the placebo effect.

The use of placebos also helps to maintain blinding. This can be made more robust by using a placebo that has been specially manufactured to cause temporary side-effects, in order to prevent the subject guessing that he or she is in the placebo arm.

Sham treatment is a term used in non-pharmacological studies, where the intervention might be a device, a psychological treatment or a physical intervention.

Placebo effect by proxy

It is not just the subject who is taking the placebo who might benefit from the placebo effect. The people around the subject, including relatives, friends and healthcare professionals, also have a strong expectation of improvement, making themselves feel better that the subject is being treated and enhancing third-party reports of clinical outcomes, even if the subject does not actually improve.

Ethical considerations

It is not always ethical to use a placebo treatment. For example, in some conditions the patient's condition can progress or health deteriorate if given a placebo.

The World Medical Association's **Declaration of Helsinki** states that the benefits, risks, burdens and effectiveness of a new intervention must be tested against those of the best current proven intervention, except in the following circumstances:

- Where no current proven intervention exists – in this case the use of a placebo (or no treatment) is acceptable.

- Where for compelling and scientifically sound methodological reasons the use of placebo is necessary to determine the efficacy or safety of an intervention and the patients who receive placebo or no treatment will not be subject to any risk of serious or irreversible harm.

Nocebo response

Whereas the placebo effect refers to the improvement experienced by a subject taking a dummy treatment, the nocebo response refers to the opposite experience, where a negative effect of an intervention is experienced because of the subject's negative beliefs and expectations about the dummy treatment. It is not due to any biochemical effect. This explains why dummy treatments, including homeopathic remedies, can have side-effects.

The side-effect profile of a real treatment in a subject can be considered to be a combination of side-effects caused by the pharmacological action of the drug and side-effects due to the nocebo response.

Scenario 8 revisited

The editor of the the Lancet *wrote back to Dr Singh. He thanked Dr Singh for submitting her case report but noted that, 'The placebo effect of co-careldopa needs to be explored and will probably explain the beneficial effects seen. To really demonstrate the efficacy of co-careldopa for pain symptoms, I would suggest a placebo-controlled double-blind strategy is more appropriate. I'll be happy to publish these results if they can be replicated in a better study.'*

TO SUMMARISE, A GOOD STUDY WILL ...

Explain the role of the placebo effect in any relationship under investigation

Describe any placebo treatment used

Discuss how blinding was maintained when a placebo was used by describing its similarity to the active treatment

Confirm that the study received ethical approval for using a placebo treatment

Scenario 9

Dr Joseph analysed the results of a trial on the usefulness of psychological interventions in patients suffering chronic pain. In one arm of the study, the patients received 20 weekly sessions with a psychologist, exploring their perceptions of pain. In the control arm, the patients were invited to chat to a nurse about their daily routine. The psychologists dramatically reduced pain scores compared with the 'placebo' intervention. Dr Joseph wrote to his Hospital Board, suggesting that sessions with psychologists were a cost-effective intervention for his patients and could reduce the need for Pain Clinic appointments.

Scenario 10

Dr Webb was amazed by the results of her trial investigating a new mood-stabilising medication for patients with bipolar disorder. Compared with patients taking lithium, the patients taking the new treatment reported fewer symptoms and they were also pleased that they did not need regular blood tests to monitor drug levels. She submitted her results to the British Journal of Psychiatry and recommended that lithium should no longer be the gold-standard treatment for patients with bipolar disorder. She hoped that her results would be the topic of the journal's editorial.

The behaviour of researchers and subjects can be influenced by what they know or believe, resulting in an observation bias. If subjects in a trial are aware of whether they are receiving a placebo or an active intervention, the answers they give can be influenced by this knowledge. Similarly, the researchers might also be influenced by any awareness of which subjects are receiving the different interventions. The behaviour of study participants and researchers can lead to bias because the subjective answers and assessments might not actually mirror the truth. This bias often occurs at a subconscious level.

Blinding, sometimes called **masking**, overcomes this problem. Treatment is regarded as 'blind' when the subject and/or the researcher do not know what trial treatments are being administered. Blinding aims to eliminate observation bias. Trial design might involve:

- **No blinding:** This occurs in an **open-label trial**.
- **Single blinding:** Either the researcher or the subject is blind to the allocation.

- **Double blinding:** The researcher and the subject are not aware of the treatment being administered. The interventions should appear identical for each treatment group.
- **Triple blinding (blind assessment):** Knowledge of the treatment is concealed from the researcher, subject and the analyst processing the results.

The blinding procedure should be clearly stated in the methodology section of the study. The groups in the trial should be treated equally as a result of blinding.

The use of placebos helps to maintain blinding. If the interventions are very different, a **double-dummy** technique can be used, in which all the subjects appear to receive both interventions (although one is a placebo), in order to maintain blinding.

Although desirable, blinding is not always possible. Open trials or single blind studies are often employed when investigating invasive or psychological interventions, for example.

The place of blinding in the study pathway is shown in **Figure 11** on page 68.

Blinding can be compromised

A study might have used blinding but that does not mean that blinding cannot be compromised. Researchers and subjects will both try to guess which arm is which. Different rates of side-effects, for example, can give the researchers and participants clues that enable them to guess correctly which treatment a subject is receiving, which can lead to an observation bias and also to subjects dropping out of the placebo arm.

Scenario 9 revisited

The Medical Director of the hospital wrote back to Dr Joseph, stating, 'It is hardly surprising that the psychotherapy patients got better. They were aware that they were getting the new intervention. While I accept that talking therapies are hard to blind, we must not rush into making costly decisions based on such trials.'

Scenario 10 revisited

Unfortunately the research article was rejected by the peer review process. The Editor of the British Journal of Psychiatry *wrote to Dr Webb, 'Unfortunately, blinding in your study was compromised because the patients taking lithium had regular blood tests. It was surely obvious who was taking lithium and who was taking the new mood-stabiliser drug. To maintain blinding and eliminate observation bias, everyone should have had the same blood tests. Sham results should have been reported for patients not taking lithium. I'm afraid that this major oversight means that I cannot publish your article.'*

TO SUMMARISE, A GOOD STUDY WILL ...

Describe how blinding was implemented

Discuss the use of placebos and other sham interventions in helping to maintain blinding

Discuss whether blinding could have been compromised

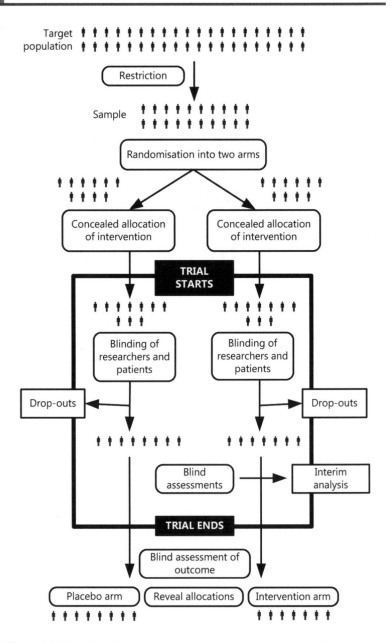

Figure 11 The study pathway

Studies report results in terms of the endpoints that were measured. There are numerous endpoints that can be used in studies, eg mortality, disease progression, disability, improvement of symptoms and quality-of-life measures.

Ideally, changes in endpoints should help doctors to make better decisions for their patients and have some clinical significance.

There are three main types of outcome used in studies – clinical, surrogate and composite.

Clinical endpoint: A measurement of a direct clinical outcome, such as mortality, morbidity or survival.

Surrogate endpoint: A measurement of an outcome used as a substitute for a clinically meaningful endpoint. The surrogate endpoint must fully capture the net effect of the intervention on the clinical endpoint. Although surrogate endpoints are believed to be predictive of important clinical outcomes, the relationship is not guaranteed. They are used because they allow effects to be measured sooner. For example, blood pressure reduction may be used as a surrogate endpoint because it is a risk factor for cerebrovascular and cardiovascular events; cardiovascular mortality, myocardial infarction, angiography or ultrasound imaging can be used as surrogate endpoints for atherosclerosis.

Surrogate markers are also used in phase 1 and phase 2 clinical trials, ie during the early stages of drug development. They can also be used in phase 3 trials, but at this stage there needs to be careful consideration of how accurately the surrogate marker reflects the clinical outcome in question and whether it will be accurate and reliable. Sample sizes for studies using surrogate markers can be smaller and the trial does not have to be as long-lasting, because changes in the surrogate endpoints usually occur before the clinical event happens.

Composite endpoint: This type of endpoint combines several measurements into a single composite endpoint, using a prespecified algorithm. This is useful when any one event occurs too infrequently to be an endpoint and it overcomes the problem of insufficient power in a study. The **primary endpoint**, ie the health characteristic that is measured in all study participants to detect a response to treatment, must be specified. Conclusions about the effectiveness of treatment should focus on this measurement. **Secondary endpoints** are other characteristics that are measured in all study participants to help describe the effects of treatment. Ideally, all the composite endpoints should be of similar importance to the patient and occur with similar frequency.

Measuring endpoints – validity and reliability

As well as specifying which endpoints were used, a study should describe how these endpoints were measured or detected. Clinical endpoints tend to be objective and easily measured, eg whether the patient died, survived or was cured. Surrogate endpoints are more widely used but are more prone to subjective assessment and differences of opinion. Problems can arise if the measurements are not made consistently.

Researchers use measuring techniques and instruments that have been shown to be valid and reliable. **Validity** refers to the extent to which a test measures what it is supposed to measure. **Reliability** refers to how consistent a test is on repeated measurements. Importantly, reliability does not imply validity.

The meaning of these two terms can be clarified by making an analogy with target practice (**Figure 12**): hitting the bull's-eye on the target is 'validity' or correctness; repeatedly hitting the same point is 'reliability' or consistency.

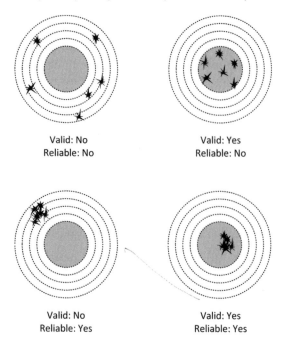

Valid: No
Reliable: No

Valid: Yes
Reliable: No

Valid: No
Reliable: Yes

Valid: Yes
Reliable: Yes

Figure 12 The relationship between validity and reliability

TO SUMMARISE, A GOOD STUDY WILL ...

Clearly state the endpoint of interest

Relate the endpoint to the clinical question

Describe how the endpoint was detected and measured

Scenario 11
Dr Harrison looked at the next research proposal submitted for ethics approval. A junior doctor wished to compare the efficacy of a new thyroxine depot injection against that of thyroxine tablets in young men with hypothyroidism. She proposed a cohort study assessing the severity of symptoms by the television viewing time of each subject at home, as hypothyroid patients tended to be tired all the time. She hypothesised that thyroxine treatment would improve hypothyroid symptoms, marked by a reduction in the amount of television viewed.

Validity refers to the extent to which a test measures what it is supposed to measure. There are many subtypes of validity. The meaning of validity in this context is not to be confused with internal and external validity (see page 5).

Types of validity

Face validity
The extent to which the test, on superficial consideration, measures what it is supposed to measure. For example, a test measuring the exercise tolerance of patients and relating it to respiratory disease severity would have face validity.

Content validity
The extent to which the test measures variables that are related to the parameter which should be measured by the test. For example, a questionnaire assessing angina severity would have content validity if the questions centred on the ability to do everyday tasks that made the heart work harder.

Criterion validity
This is used to demonstrate the accuracy of a measure or procedure by comparing it with another measure or procedure that has been demonstrated to be valid. Criterion validity can be concurrent or predictive.

- **Concurrent validity:** The extent to which the test correlates with a measure that has been previously validated. For example, a score on a rating scale for pain would have concurrent validity if it agreed with a previously validated rating scale.

- **Predictive validity:** The extent to which the test is able to predict something it should theoretically be able to predict. For example, a written examination would have predictive validity if it measured performance in secondary school and successfully predicted employment status in adulthood.

Construct validity

The extent to which the test measures a theoretical construct by a specific measuring device or procedure. For example, an IQ test would have construct validity if its results reflected the theoretical concept of intelligence. Constructive validity can be convergent or divergent.

- **Convergent validity:** The extent to which the test is similar to other tests that are measuring the same construct. For example, a digital thermometer would have convergent validity with a mercury-based thermometer if it returned similar results.

- **Divergent (discriminant) validity:** The extent to which the test is not similar to other tests that are measuring different constructs. For example, a postgraduate assessment of critical appraisal skills of doctors would have discriminant validity if it returned results dissimilar to a multiple-choice question paper testing knowledge of diseases.

Incremental validity

The extent to which the test provides a significant improvement in addition to the use of another approach. A test has incremental validity if it helps more than if it were not used. For example, ultrasound scanning gives better estimates of fetal gestation age than clinical examination alone.

Scenario 11 revisited

Dr Harrison wrote back to the young researcher, stating that, 'Selecting patients and assessing them on the basis of their viewing habits seems inappropriate to me. Hypothyroid patients might do many things apart from increase their television viewing time (and I'm not even sure about that!), so it appears to me that a more valid assessment method is required.'

TO SUMMARISE, A GOOD STUDY WILL ...

Describe what was measured and how this related to the endpoints

Scenario 12

Dr Nolan was supervising a class of first-year medical students. All the students were asked to take each other's blood pressure until they were comfortable using a sphygmomanometer. Dr Nolan noticed that, halfway through the session, some of the students looked bemused. He asked one student what the matter was. 'It's these sphygmomanometers,' said the student, 'They never give the same result twice!' After the session, Dr Nolan wrote to the Clinical Tutor, suggesting that an investment be made in better equipment.

Studies often involve the measurement of one or more variables. Good research technique involves commenting on the reliability of these measurements, ie the consistency of test results on repeat measurements. Repeat measurements can be by the same person, by more than one person and/or across time:

- **Intrarater reliability:** This looks at the level of agreement between assessments by one rater of the same material at two or more different times.

- **Inter-rater reliability:** This measures the level of agreement between assessments made by two or more raters at the same time.

- **Test–retest reliability:** This refers to the level of agreement between the initial test results and the results of repeat measurements made at a later date.

Good reliability ensures consistency of the results being achieved and of the conclusions that are being drawn from the study.

Internal consistency

If a scale has several questions or items which all address the same issue, then we usually expect each individual to get similar scores for those questions. **Crohnbach's alpha** (α) is used to assess this internal consistency. If Cronbach's α is ≥ 0.5 there is moderate agreement and if Crohnbach's α is ≥ 0.8 there is excellent agreement.

Continuous data

Reliability both within individuals and between observers can be quantified in several different ways:

- If the size of the differences between repeated measurements is of interest, the **Bland–Altman limits of agreement** can be used. The difference between each pair of scores is plotted on the vertical axis versus their mean on the horizontal axis. Perfect agreement is shown by the points lying on the horizontal line through the zero value. Poorer level of agreement is shown by points lying further away from the horizontal line.

- If a relative summary is of interest, then the **coefficient of variation** might be useful.

- The **intraclass correlation coefficient** is also sometimes used. This is for use with tests measuring quantitative variables. It describes the extent to which two continuous measures taken by different people or two measurements taken by the same person on different occasions are related. This can be useful for comparing the repeatability of several measures. However, it gives no indication of absolute differences.

Categorical data

To assess the level of agreement for data that fall into categories, Cohen's kappa is used.

The **kappa statistic** (κ), also known as 'Cohen's statistic' or the 'chance-corrected proportional agreement statistic', measures the level of agreement between assessments made by two or more raters at the same time where responses can fall into categories. This is also known as **inter-rater reliability**.

Measurements can agree purely by chance. The kappa statistic indicates the level of the agreement between measurements by different raters and gives an indication as to whether this agreement is more than could be expected by chance. If agreement is no more than expected by chance, then $\kappa = 0$. With perfect agreement, $\kappa = 1$ (**Table 8**). To avoid low kappa values, measurements by researchers can be improved by simply agreeing criteria and measurement conditions. One disadvantage of this measurement of agreement is that it is sensitive to the prevalence / proportion of individuals in each group.

To calculate kappa:

$$\kappa = (P_O - P_E) / (1 - P_E)$$

where:

P_O = observed agreement

P_E = agreement expected by chance

KAPPA	STRENGTH OF AGREEMENT
0	Chance agreement only
0.01–0.20	Poor agreement beyond chance
0.21–0.40	Fair agreement beyond chance
0.41–0.60	Moderate agreement beyond chance
0.61–0.80	Good agreement beyond chance
0.81–0.99	Very good agreement beyond chance
1.0	Perfect agreement

Table 8 Kappa (κ) and the strength of agreement

A **weighted kappa** takes account of how far apart any disagreements are.

Other types of reliability

Alternative-form reliability
This describes reliability of similar forms of the test, looking at the same material either at the same time or immediately consecutively. For example, the temperature reading from a mercury thermometer can be compared with that from a digital thermometer.

Split-half reliability
This describes the reliability of a test that is divided in two, with each half being used to assess the same material under similar circumstances.

Scenario 12 revisited

The Clinical Tutor wrote back to Dr Nolan, thanking him for his feedback. He went on, 'The issue of reliability is indeed an important one in blood pressure measurements. I don't think simply having a new set of sphygmomanometers will make much of a difference, however, because the reliability of the measure is never going to be perfect, no matter who uses the sphygmomanometer!'

TO SUMMARISE, A GOOD STUDY WILL ...

Provide evidence that measuring instruments are reliable, usually by referring to earlier studies

Quote correlation coefficient values

Describe how reliability was improved by training and standardisation

SECTION C

INTERPRETING RESULTS

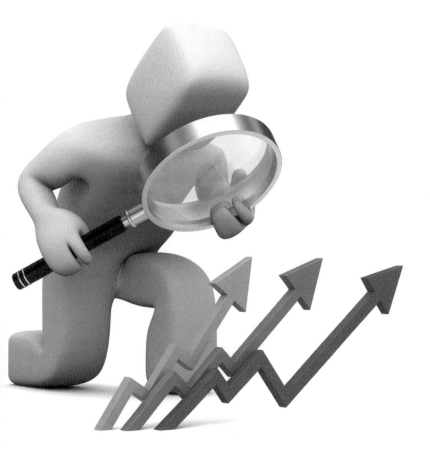

Statistics is the mathematical science of collecting, organising, analysing, presenting and interpreting data.

Descriptive versus inferential statistics

Descriptive statistics
Used to organise or summarise data collected from a sample population. For example, there might be a table in the results section of a clinical paper which summarises the baseline characteristics of subjects in the different treatment arms.

Inferential statistics
Uses data collected from a sample population to make generalisations about the target population from which the sample population was drawn.

Variables, attributes and parameters

Variable
Any entity that can take on different values. Examples include sample size, gender, age and drug dosage. Variables can be **qualitative** or **quantitative** values.

Two further terms are used when describing relationships:

- An **independent variable** is manipulated in the study. It is also known as the 'experimental' variable.
- A **dependent variable** is affected by the change in the value of the independent variable. It is also known as the 'outcome' variable.

Attribute
A specific value of a variable. For example, gender has two attributes, male and female.

Parameter
Any numerical quantity that characterises a population. For example, the mean and the standard deviation are two parameters that characterise a normal distribution.

Accuracy versus precision
- **Accuracy:** How close the measurement is to its true value.
- **Precision:** How close repeat measurements are to each other.

Ideally, a measurement is accurate and precise but this isn't always the case. A result can often be very accurate but not precise or vice versa.

EPIDEMIOLOGICAL DATA

Epidemiology is the scientific study of the distribution, causes and control of diseases in populations. Studies frequently provide epidemiological data to describe the disease or population of interest.

There are two main measures of disease frequency, **incidence** and **prevalence**.

Incidence

Incidence: The rate of occurrence of new cases over a period of time in a defined population (**Figure 13**). It is a measure of the risk of disease.

$$incidence = \frac{\text{number of new cases over a period of time}}{\text{population size}}$$

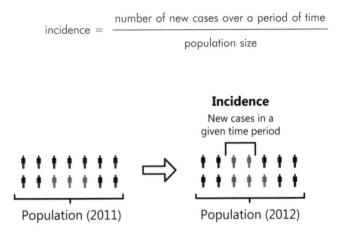

Figure 13 Incidence

The incidence can be given as a **crude rate**, which is the rate that applies to the whole population without any adjustment. A **specific rate** can be given, which only applies to a subgroup in the population.

- **Mortality rate:** This is a type of incidence rate that expresses the risk of death over a period of time in a population.

$$\text{mortality rate} = \frac{\text{number of deaths over a period of time}}{\text{population size}}$$

- **Standardised mortality rate:** The mortality rate is adjusted to compensate for a confounder, for example age.

- **Standardised mortality ratio:** The ratio of the observed standardised mortality rate (from the study population) to the expected standardised mortality rate (from the standard population). The reference value is 100. Converting a mortality rate into a ratio makes it easier to compare different populations. The lower the ratio, the better.

- **Hospital standardised mortality ratio (HSMR):** A measure of overall mortality in hospitals, used in conjunction with other indicators to assess quality of care. The HSMR is adjusted for many factors, including sex, age, socioeconomic deprivation, diagnosis and method of patient admission to hospital.

In 2009 a report by the Healthcare Commission detailed a catalogue of failings at Mid Staffordshire NHS Foundation Trust which were only uncovered when unusually high mortality rates at the hospital triggered alerts[1]. The HSMR for the hospital for 2005/06 was 127, meaning that 27% more patients died than might be expected. It was estimated that, between 2005 and 2008, 400 more people died at the hospital than would be expected. The Chairman of the Trust resigned, the Chief Executive was suspended and an independent inquiry was launched.

1   Investigation into Mid Staffordshire NHS Foundation Trust: Commission for Healthcare Audit and Inspection, March 2009 ISBN 978-1-84562-220-6.

- **Morbidity rate:** This is the rate of occurrence of new non-fatal cases of the disease in a defined population at risk over a given time period.

$$\text{morbidity rate} = \frac{\text{number of new non-fatal cases over a period of time}}{\text{size of population at risk}}$$

- **Standardised morbidity rate:** The morbidity rate is adjusted to compensate for a confounder.

- **Standardised morbidity ratio:** Ratio of the observed standardised morbidity rate (from the study population) to the expected standardised morbidity rate (from the standard population).

Prevalence

Point prevalence: The proportion of a defined population having the disease at a given point in time (**Figure 14**). Prevalence is useful for planning health services.

$$\text{point prevalence} = \frac{\text{number of people with the disease at a given time}}{\text{size of population at the same time}}$$

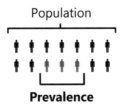

Population

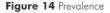

Prevalence

Figure 14 Prevalence

Incidence and prevalence are related by the following equation

$$\text{prevalence at any time point} = \text{incidence} \times \text{average duration of the disease}$$

Period prevalence: The proportion of a population that has the disease during a given time period (such as annual prevalence).

$$\text{period prevalence} = \frac{\text{number of people with the disease or developing the disease in a period of time}}{\text{size of population at the same time}}$$

Lifetime prevalence: This is the proportion of a population that either has or has had the disease at a given point in time.

Self-assessment exercise 8

1. A cohort study was carried out on 200 men. Half of the participants had been exposed to passive smoking while working in pubs. The other half of the participants had not been exposed to passive smoking. After 10 years, there were four cases of lung cancer in the exposed group and one case in the unexposed group. What is the annual incidence rate of lung cancer in the exposed group? What is the annual incidence rate in the unexposed group? What is the overall annual incidence rate?

2. The incidence of cystic fibrosis is 1 in 2500 births. How many new cases will a paediatrician expect to see over 10 years if the hospital she works in delivers 90 babies a month?

3. The annual mortality rate for acute pancreatitis is 1.3 per 100 000. If there are 60 million people in the UK, how many deaths from acute pancreatitis are expected every week?

4. 85 000 people in the UK have multiple sclerosis. What is the prevalence rate per 100 000 of the population if the UK population is 60 million people?

5. Assuming the population size is unchanged, what will happen to the prevalence of a disease if there is:

   a. Immigration of cases into the area?

   b. Emigration of cases out of the area?

   c. Immigration of healthy people into the area?

   d. An increase in the case fatality rate?

Scenario 13

Dr Wilson returned from his lunch break with renewed vigour. He had just read the conclusion of a trial on the treatment of ear infections in 1000 children using a new antibiotic, zapitillin, compared with his usual choice, amoxicillin. In the zapitillin arm, 240 out of 300 children who completed the study improved (80%). In the amoxicillin arm, 300 out of 400 children who completed the study improved (75%). He sent a copy of the paper to his colleague, proposing that zapitillin be the first-choice antibiotic in the hospital formulary.

In most studies some of the individuals who are eligible and participate in a trial do not make it to the end of the trial. There are many reasons why such **drop-outs** occur, including early deaths, loss to follow-up (individuals who cannot be contacted or who have moved out of the study area), voluntary withdrawal from the trial, non-compliance with the trial conditions and ineligible patients. Some individuals might also not be able to take the treatments offered to them in the trial. Ideally, a research paper should account for all its subjects who were eligible and started the trial, explaining the reasons why some did not finish the trial. This is sometimes depicted in a flow diagram or table.

Success rates can vary widely depending on which figures are used. Determining the sample of patients to be analysed is a key step in reporting clinical trials.

Per-protocol analysis

A per-protocol or on-treatment analysis is an approach used in which data from only those subjects who received treatment and complied with the trial protocol through to completion are considered in the analysis. Subjects who did not complete the trial protocol are not accounted for when calculating success rates.

The advantage of this **explanatory approach** is that it gives a good insight into how things might be if processes are completed and gives an indication of the true effect of a treatment. The disadvantage of this method is that it can introduce bias related to excluding participants from analysis (attrition or exclusion bias). If these subjects are not accounted for in the analysis of the results, the results and conclusions can be misleading and important effects of the intervention (eg intolerable side-effects) can be lost.

Intention-to-treat analysis

In an **intention-to-treat analysis** all the study participants allocated are included in the analyses as part of the groups to which they are allocated, regardless of whether they completed the study or not. It keeps them in the original groups for the purpose of statistical analysis.

A per-protocol analysis tends to enhance any difference between the different groups in a study whereas an intention-to-treat analysis tends to produce more conservative results. The intention-to-treat method is also known as the **pragmatic approach**. Success rates based on intention-to-treat analyses tend to mirror the results seen in real-life practice.

The intention-to-treat analysis is usually considered as the analysis of choice and, if necessary, the study could have a secondary analysis done using the per-protocol approach.

Handling missing data

Steps to achieve an intention-to-treat analysis should be considered in both the design and conduct of a trial. Any eligibility errors can be avoided by careful inspection before random allocation. Efforts should be made to ensure minimal drop-outs from treatment and losses to follow-up. In some studies, an active run-in phase is introduced at the start of the study and this can help identify patients who are likely to drop out.

During the trial, continuing clinical support should be available to all participants.

If drop-outs occur in a study, the researcher has to decide how to include these individuals in an intention-to-treat analysis. With luck, some data will have been collected up to the point at which these subjects left the trial. Ideally, data on the primary endpoints are collected after drop out.

- In **last observation carried forward**, the last recorded results of individuals who drop out are carried forward to the end of the trial and incorporated into the final analysis of the results.

- In a **worst-case scenario** analysis, subjects who drop out are treated as non-responders and recorded as having the worst outcome possible. This is the most cautious and pessimistic approach.

- In **imputation**, missing data are substituted to allow the data analysis to proceed. For example, plausible values from similar but complete records can be used to fill in missing values. This is called 'hot-deck imputation'. There are other techniques available. The analysis should take into account the greater degree of uncertainty that is caused by imputation.

- In a **sensitivity analysis**, assumptions are made when the missing values are put in. Sensitivity analyses can also be carried out to include different scenarios of assumptions, such as the worst-case and best-case scenarios. Worst-case scenario sensitivity analysis is performed by assigning the worst outcomes to the missing patients in the group who show the best results. These results are then compared with the initial analysis, which excludes the missing data.

- In studies that have many drop-outs, the **drop-out event** itself should be considered as an important endpoint.

It is important to establish whether the reasons drop-outs are no longer taking part are in some way attributable to the intervention. The chance of there being drop-outs should be minimised early on when the study is being planned and during trial monitoring.

The use of 'last observation carried forward' can lead to underestimation or overestimation of treatment effects. **Figure 15** shows the result of treating a depressed patient with an antidepressant. Over the trial, the patient's depressive symptoms improve gradually, so that at the end of the trial they were less depressed than at the start.

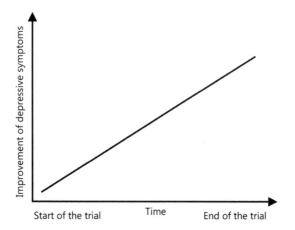

Figure 15 The result of treating a depressed patient with an antidepressant

If a different individual dropped out of the study at an early stage and the last observation was carried forward, the results could underestimate the true effect of the antidepressant, which would have been apparent had the individual completed the trial (**Figure 16**). The risk of making a type 2 error is increased (see page 124).

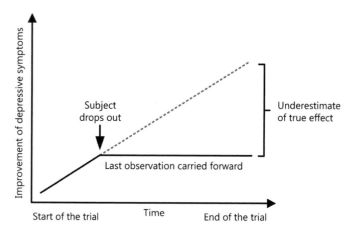

Figure 16 Underestimation of a treatment effect

Overestimation of a treatment effect can occur with 'last observation carried forward' in conditions that normally deteriorate with time. **Figure 17** shows the results of the Mini Mental State Examination (MMSE) score of a dementing individual who is being treated with an anti-dementia drug. Over the trial, their dementia will progress, but at a slower rate with treatment.

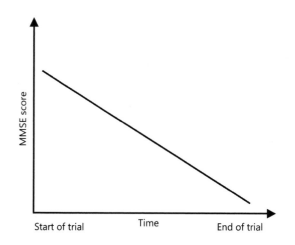

Figure 17 Decline in the Mini Mental State Examination (MMSE) score

If a different individual drops out of the trial at an early stage, the effects of the anti-dementia drug in delaying the progression of dementia might be overstated (**Figure 18**). The risk of making a type 1 error is increased (see page 123).

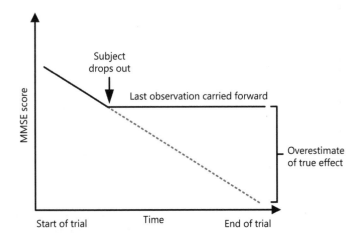

Figure 18 Overestimation of a treatment effect

Scenario 13 revisited

Dr Wilson's colleague read the paper too, but came to a different conclusion. He emailed Dr Wilson, 'I disagree with the conclusions the researchers have drawn. Five hundred patients were enrolled into each arm of the study. I worked out that the results did not take into account the drop-outs in both arms. Intention-to-treat analysis shows that amoxicillin gave better results, with 300 out of 500 children improving (60%). In contrast, only 240 children improved with zapitillin (48%). I won't be prescribing zapitillin unless the child has an allergy to amoxicillin, but thanks for drawing my attention to the paper.'

RISKS AND ODDS

Risk: In clinical research, risk has the same meaning as probability. Risk is the probability of something happening. Risk is the number of times an event is likely to occur divided by the total number of events possible. It is expressed as P and is presented either as a number between 0 and 1 or as a percentage:

If 1 out of 6 people fall ill, the risk of falling ill is $1/6 = 0.167 = 16.7\%$

Odds: Odds is also another way of expressing chance. The odds is the ratio of the number of times an event is likely to occur divided by the number of times it is likely not to occur. This is expressed as a ratio or fraction:

If 1 out of 6 people fall ill, the odds of falling ill is $1/5 = 0.2$

Contingency tables

When comparing risks and odds across two groups, the first step is to tabulate the study results in a contingency table, also known as a 2 × 2 table (**Table 9**). The contingency table consists of rows and columns of cells. Cells a, b, c and d are the 2 × 2 table; the other cells help to make sense of the table.

Contingency tables can be a source of confusion because there are different ways of displaying the same information. Always maintain a consistent approach by having the exposure (to a risk factor or intervention) across the rows and the outcome event status down the columns. The 'outcome event' always refers to the worst outcome, such as death.

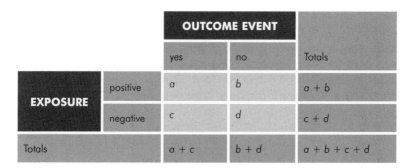

Table 9 Generic 2 × 2 contingency table

Example 1: In a cohort study, 100 subjects are exposed to cigarette smoking and 75 subjects are not exposed to smoking. At the end of the study, 27 subjects in the smoking group developed cancer. Only four subjects in the non-smoking group developed cancer.

The steps to complete a 2 × 2 table (see **Table 10**) are:

- The rows are labelled 'smoking' (exposure), positive or negative.
- The columns are labelled 'cancer' (worst outcome event), yes or no.
- 100 subjects were exposed to cigarette smoking so $a + b = 100$.
- 75 subjects were not exposed to smoking, so $c + d = 75$.
- In the smoking group, 27 subjects developed the worst outcome, so $a = 27$.
- In the non-smoking group, four subjects developed the worst outcome, so $c = 4$.
- $b = 100 - 27 = 73$ subjects developed the best outcome in the smoking group.
- $d = 75 - 4 = 71$ subjects developed the best outcome in the non-smoking group.

		CANCER		
		yes	no	Totals
SMOKING	positive	27 (a)	73 (b)	100
	negative	4 (c)	71 (d)	75
Totals		31	144	175

Table 10 Completed 2 × 2 contingency table for **Example 1**

Some studies will report the best outcome figures. Care needs to be exercised so that the 2 × 2 table is completed correctly.

Example 2: In a randomised controlled trial of an analgesic, 28/37 subjects improved on the new treatment and 12/30 subjects improved in the placebo arm.

The steps to complete a 2 × 2 table (see **Table 11**) are:

- The rows are labelled 'new treatment' (exposure), positive or negative.
- The columns are labelled 'pain' (worst outcome event), yes or no.
- 37 subjects were exposed to the new treatment, so $a + b = 37$.
- 30 subjects were not exposed to the new treatment, so $c + d = 30$.
- In the treatment group, nine subjects $(37 - 28)$ developed the worst outcome, so $a = 9$.
- In the placebo group, 18 subjects $(30 - 12)$ developed the worst outcome, so $c = 18$.
- $b = 37 - 9 = 28$ people developed the best outcome in the treatment group.
- $d = 30 - 18 = 12$ developed the best outcome in the placebo arm.

		PAIN		
		yes	no	Totals
NEW TREATMENT	positive	9 (a)	28 (b)	37
	negative	18 (c)	12 (d)	30
Totals		27	40	67

Table 11 Completed 2 × 2 contingency table for **Example 2**

Other aspects of risk can be derived from the 2×2 contingency table (**Table 12**).

	FORMULA
Control event rate (CER) (outcome event rate in control group)	$\dfrac{c}{c + d}$
Experimental event rate (EER) (outcome event rate in experimental group)	$\dfrac{a}{a + b}$
Absolute risk reduction (ARR)	$CER - EER$
Relative risk (RR)	$\dfrac{EER}{CER}$
Relative risk reduction (RRR)	$\dfrac{CER - EER}{CER}$
Numbers needed to treat (NNT)	$\dfrac{1}{ARR}$
Odds of outcome in exposed group	$\dfrac{a}{b}$
Odds of outcome in non-exposed group	$\dfrac{c}{d}$
Odds ratio	$\dfrac{a / b}{c / d} = \dfrac{ad}{bc}$

Table 12 Derivation of other aspects of risk from the 2×2 contingency table

Absolute risk

Absolute risk is the incidence rate of the outcome. Remember that the outcome is the worst outcome.

control event rate (CER) = risk in subjects not exposed = $\dfrac{c}{c+d}$

experimental event rate (EER) = risk in subjects exposed = $\dfrac{a}{a+b}$

Absolute risk reduction

The absolute risk reduction (ARR) is the drop in risk going from the control group to the experimental group:

absolute risk reduction = CER − EER

The absolute risk reduction is also known as the **absolute benefit increase** (ABI).

Relative risk

The relative risk (RR) or 'risk ratio' is the ratio of the risk of the outcome in the experimental group to the risk of the outcome in the control group.

relative risk = $\dfrac{EER}{CER}$

- If the relative risk is equal to 1, there is **no risk difference** between the groups.
- If the relative risk is greater than 1, there is an **increased risk** of the outcome in the experimental arm.
- If the relative risk is less than 1, there is a **reduced risk** of the outcome in the experimental arm.

Note that absolute risks are more useful than relative risks. Relative risk values can be large and impressive even when the underlying absolute risk reductions are very small. See **Figure 19** for an example.

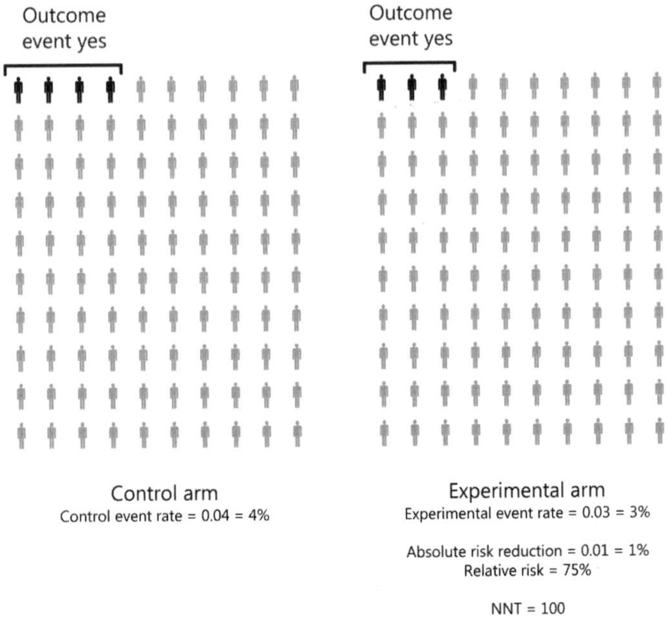

Figure 19 An impressive relative risk figure but very small absolute risk values

Relative risk reduction

Relative risk reduction (RRR) is the proportional reduction in rates of outcomes between control and experimental subjects in a study:

$$\text{relative risk reduction} = \frac{CER - EER}{CER}$$

The relative risk reduction is also known as the **relative benefit increase** (RBI).

- If the CER = 0.8 and the EER = 0.4, then the RRR = 50% (risk reduces by 50% of the CER risk).
- If the CER = 0.8 and the EER = 0.6, then the RRR = 25% (risk reduces by 25% of the CER risk).

Number needed to treat

The number needed to treat (NNT) is the number of subjects who must be treated with the intervention, compared with the control, for one additional subject to experience the beneficial outcome. It is the reciprocal of the absolute risk reduction between two interventions. The lower the value of NNT the better. The minimum value for NNT is 1; the maximum value is infinity.

$$\text{number needed to treat} = \frac{1}{ARR}$$

- If NNT = 8, for every eight patients in the experimental arm, one additional person gets the beneficial outcome.

NNTs are easy to interpret but comparisons between NNTs can only be made if the baseline risks are the same. There is no cut-off level for guidance.

The NNH is the **number needed to harm**. This is the number of subjects treated for one extra subject to have the adverse outcome, compared with the control intervention. Smaller NNH values are worse (ie harm is more frequent).

NNTs and NNHs should be reported as whole numbers. NNTs should be rounded up to the next whole number and NNHs should be rounded down.

The NNH:NNT ratio is indicative of the risk/benefit ratio.

Odds ratio

Odds ratio (OR) is an alternative way of comparing how likely outcomes are between two groups.

The odds ratio is the ratio of the odds of having the outcome in the experimental group relative to the odds of having the outcome in the control group.

It is used in cross-sectional studies and case–control studies. In a case–control study, the exposure is often the presence or absence of a risk factor for a disease, and the outcome is the presence or absence of the disease.

$$\text{odds ratio} = \frac{ad}{bc}$$

- An odds ratio of 1.0 (or unity) reflects exactly the same outcome rates in both groups, ie **no effect**.
- An odds ratio greater than 1 indicates that the estimated likelihood of developing the outcome is **greater** among those in the experimental arm.
- An odds ratio less than 1 indicates that the estimated likelihood of developing the outcome is **less** among those in the experimental arm.

If a 'log odds ratio' is given in the clinical paper, remember that a log odds ratio of zero reflects the same outcome rates in both groups, not the value 1.

Interpreting negative results

If the 2 × 2 table is formatted as recommended above, with the outcome event being the worst outcome possible, some results may be negative numbers. Negative results are interpreted as follows:

A *negative* absolute risk reduction is interpreted as an **absolute risk increase**.

- Absolute risk reduction = −0.5 is an absolute risk increase = 0.5

A *negative* relative risk reduction is interpreted as a **relative risk increase**.

- Relative risk reduction = −0.3 is a relative risk increase = 0.3

A *negative* number needed to treat is interpreted as a **number needed to harm**.

- Number needed to treat = −4 is a number needed to harm = 4
  ie there is one additional harmful outcome for every 4 patients.

Self-assessment exercise 9

1. In a group of 60 patients treated with diclofenac sodium, 10 complained of indigestion. What are the risk and odds of developing this side-effect in this group?

2. In a group of 220 patients with heart disease, the risk of death in the first year is 5%. How many patients will die in the first year?

3. In a cohort study, 100 patients were followed up for 20 years. At the start, 56 of the patients had been exposed to asbestos. At the end of the study, of those exposed to asbestos, 20 had lung disease. Of those not exposed, only two had lung disease. Tabulate this information in a contingency table. Calculate the control event rate (CER) and the experimental event rate (EER). Calculate the odds of the outcome in the exposed group and the odds of the outcome in the non-exposed group.

4. A total of 2000 patients with fungal nail infections were randomly allocated to a new topical treatment or placebo (in equal numbers). A total of 66 patients in the placebo group had another infection within 1 month, compared with 21 patients in the treated group. Draw a 2 × 2 table for this information and calculate the following: absolute risk in the treated group (EER), absolute risk in the untreated group (CER), the relative risk (RR), the relative risk reduction (RRR), the absolute risk reduction (ARR) and the number needed to treat (NNT).

5. In a study, 17 patients treated with a new analgesic reported a significant improvement in pain symptoms, whereas four patients did not. In a control group treated with paracetamol, only one of the 20 patients reported a benefit. Calculate the control event rate (CER), the experimental event rate (EER) and the odds ratio (OR).

TYPES OF DATA

Data can be classified as either qualitative or quantitative.

Qualitative data

Qualitative data are also known as **categorical** or **non-numerical** data.

Examples of qualitative data:

- Gender: male, female
- Marital status: single, married, divorced, widowed
- Colour: red, yellow, blue, silver, green
- Outcome: cured, not cured

If there are only two possible attributes for a categorical variable, the term **binary data** can be used. The term **multicategory data** is used when there are more than two possible categories.

Quantitative data

Quantitative data are also known as **numerical** data and are classified as either discrete or continuous.

Discrete data have a finite number of possible values and tend to be made up of integers (or whole numbers). Counts are examples of discrete data:

- Number of pupils absent each day at school: 7, 3, 13, 14, 4
- Waiting time to see a doctor in days: 2, 1, 3, 2, 4, 2, 1.

Continuous data have infinite possibilities. Continuous data values can include decimal places:

- Diameter of tumours: 1.23 cm, 1.78 cm, 2.25 cm
- Weight of patients: 67.234 kg, 89.935 kg, 101.563 kg

Quantitative data can be converted into categorical data by using cut-off points (see **Table 13**). Results of rating scales are often converted into cured/not-cured categories. This is because categorical data are easier to tabulate and analyse. However, the conversion means some data are discarded and it gets harder to detect a statistically significant difference.

BLOOD PRESSURE (QUANTITATIVE DATA)		BLOOD PRESSURE (CATEGORIES)
80/30 mmHg		Hypotensive
120/70 mmHg		Normotensive
145/85 mmHg	⇨	Normotensive
160/85 mmHg		Normotensive
150/100 mmHg		Hypertensive
165/105 mmHg		Hypertensive

Table 13 Converting quantitative data to categorical data

Measuring instruments and data collection

The measuring instrument used to measure data will determine the type of data collected:

- Fun weighing machine – results given as 'skinny', 'normal', 'fat', 'too fat' (qualitative data)
- Digital weighing machine – results given in kg to two decimal places (quantitative continuous data)

MEASURING DATA

A scale of measurement is used to assign a value to a variable. There are four types of measurement scales, listed below in order of increasing complexity. The measurement scale determines the types of statistics that can be used to analyse the data.

Nominal scales

A nominal scale is organised in categories which have no inherent order and which bear no mathematical relationship to each other. A nominal scale simply labels objects, eg:

- Gender: male, female
- Hair colour: blond, brunette, brown, black, ginger

Ordinal scales

An ordinal scale is organised in categories that have an inherent order or rank. The categories are not given a numerical value, so the interval between categories is not meaningful, eg:

- Social class: I, II, III, IV, V
- Severity of disease: mild, moderate, severe

Interval scales

An interval scale is organised in a meaningful way, with the differences between points being equal across the scale. Interval data have no true starting point. The value zero on an interval scale has no special meaning; it is simply another point of measurement on the scale.

- The Celsius temperature scale is an example of an interval scale: 0°C does not mean there is no temperature, as minus temperatures are possible too. Also, although 80°C is as different from 40°C as 40°C is from 0°C, it does not mean that 80°C is twice the temperature of 40°C, as the scale does not start at 0°C.

Ratio scales

A ratio scale is the same as an interval scale but there is a true zero. There is no number below zero.

- The Kelvin temperature scale is an example of a ratio scale: 0 K means there is no temperature as it signifies that all thermal motion has ceased. Also, 80 K is as different from 40 K as 40 K is from 0 K and 80 K is twice the temperature of 40 K.

Using scales

Qualitative data tend to be measured on nominal or ordinal scales. Quantitative data tend to be measured on interval or ratio scales.

Nominal and ordinal data can be analysed with non-parametric statistics. Interval and ratio data can be analysed using parametric statistics.

Table 14 summarises the features of the different types of scales.

	NOMINAL	ORDINAL	INTERVAL	RATIO
Shows a difference	Yes	Yes	Yes	Yes
Shows direction of difference	—	Yes	Yes	Yes
Shows amount of difference	—	—	Yes	Yes
Has an absolute zero	—	—	—	Yes

Table 14 Measurement scales.
Adapted from www.webster.edu/~woolflm/statwhatis.html

Self-assessment exercise 10

1. What data type and scale are appropriate for each of the variables?

    a. The diagnosis of patients on a ward

    b. The sex of patients

    c. The weight of patients

    d. The staging of cancer

    e. The age of patients

    f. The ethnicity of patients

    g. The blood cholesterol level

    h. Patient blood groups

    i. Body temperature

    j. Marital status

    k. Education level

After data are collected, the information needs to be organised and summarised. Patterns or trends might emerge and this can help determine which statistical analyses should be performed on the data.

A **probability distribution** links all the possible values of a random variable in an experiment with the likelihood of the occurrence of each of these values.

- A coin is tossed once. The outcome can be heads or tails. The probability of getting no heads is 0.5. The probability of getting one head is 0.5. This information displayed in a table would constitute a probability distribution.

Number of heads	Probability
0	0.5
1	0.5

- A coin is tossed twice. Each time the coin is tossed the outcome can be head or tail. The probability of getting no heads is 0.25. The probability of getting one head is 0.5. The probability of getting two heads is 0.25. This information displayed in a table would constitute a probability distribution.

Number of heads	Probability
0	0.25
1	0.5
2	0.25

Depending on whether a random variable is discrete or continuous, the probability distribution can be **discrete** or **continuous**.

The examples of tossing a coin are discrete distributions. It is only possible to get whole numbers of heads. For example, it is not possible to get 1.5 heads. Discrete probability distributions can be shown in tabular form.

A continuous variable generates a continuous probability distribution. This type of distribution is best shown in a graphical format or expressed as an equation or formula.

There are three common probability distributions to consider:

- Binomial (discrete)
- Poisson (discrete)
- Normal (continuous)

Binomial distribution

In a **binomial experiment** there are a fixed number of runs in which a random variable can have two possible outcomes, the probabilities of which are the same in each run. Each run is independent. The outcome of each run does not affect the outcome of other runs.

The **binomial distribution** is the probability distribution of a binomial random variable. Tossing a coin five times and calculating the probabilities of getting from zero to five heads is an example of a binomial distribution.

The **Bernoulli distribution** is a special case of the binomial distribution in which an experiment on a variable with only two possible outcomes is run just once. Tossing a coin once and determining the likelihood of getting a head is an example of a Bernoulli distribution.

Poisson distribution

In a **Poisson experiment** there are repeated runs in which a random variable can have two possible outcomes. The mean number of outcomes that occur in a period of continuous space or time is known. The number of runs is not fixed.

The **Poisson distribution** can be used to determine the probability of getting an outcome in a Poisson experiment. For example, knowing that, on average, five babies are born every day on a maternity ward, one can calculate the likelihood that exactly six babies will be born tomorrow or the likelihood that fewer than three babies will be born tomorrow.

Normal distribution

The normal probability distribution is a continuous variable distribution. A majority of biological measures have an approximately normal distribution.

The normal distribution has many convenient mathematical properties. It has a characteristic bell-shaped distribution that is symmetrical about its mean value. This means that the mean is the same as the median and the mode. The normal distribution can be described completely by its mean and variance.

Central limit theorem

This is a theorem that states that the sum of a large number of random variables is distributed approximately normally, no matter what the probability distribution of the original variables. This theorem allows the use of the normal distribution in creating confidence intervals and for hypothesis testing. It allows us to estimate the standard error (see pages 117–119) from a single sample.

Reference ranges

These are a range of values or an interval which contains the values obtained from the majority of a sample of normal people. The normal distribution can be useful in calculating the reference ranges because of its unique properties.

DESCRIBING CATEGORICAL DATA

Categorical data (mode, frequency)

The **mode** is the most common value:

- A **unimodal distribution** has a single peak.
- A **bimodal distribution** has two modal values. This type of distribution can be seen if two types of data are mixed, eg the heights of a group of men and women.

The **frequency** is the number of values in each category. For example, in **Table 13** on page 101, the mode is 'normotensive' and the frequencies are:

- Hypotensive (1 observation)
- Normotensive (3 observations)
- Hypertensive (2 observations)

Presenting the frequencies as proportions is more useful than simply knowing the absolute frequency in each category. For example, 50% normotensive cases is more useful than knowing there were three normotensive observations. Ideally, the absolute numbers and proportions should be given together because the absolute frequencies are still needed for statistical analyses.

Normally distributed data (mean, standard deviation)

A normal distribution, also known as a 'Gaussian distribution', is a perfectly symmetrical, bell-shaped curve, as shown in **Figure 20**.

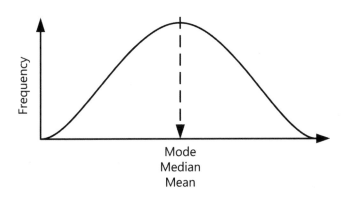

Mode
Median
Mean

Figure 20 Normal distribution

Mean: The sum of all the values divided by the number of values.

$$\text{mean} = \frac{\text{sum of all the values}}{\text{the number of values}}$$

$$\bar{x} = \frac{\Sigma x}{n}$$

The mean uses all the data and is easy to calculate. However, it is not robust to aberrant values and can be difficult to interpret.

In a perfect normal distribution, the mean, median and mode are of equal value and lie in the centre of the distribution.

Weighted mean: In situations where some values of the variable are more important than other values, a weight can be attached to each value to reflect the relative importance of each value. If the weight is equal across all the values, the weighted mean is equal to the arithmetic mean.

Variance: The dispersion of values around the mean is indicated by the variance. This is equal to the average distance by which each individual observation differs from the mean value.

The variance is the sum of all the differences between all the values and the mean, squared and divided by the total number of observations minus 1 (the degrees of freedom):

$$\text{variance } (v) = \frac{\sum (x - \bar{x})^2}{n - 1}$$

Standard deviation (SD): A statistical measure that describes the degree of data spread about the mean – the amount the values will deviate from the mean. It is a measure of precision. It has the same units as the observations.

Standard deviation is calculated as the square root of the variance:

$$\text{standard deviation} = \sqrt{v} = \sqrt{\frac{\sum (x - \bar{x})^2}{n - 1}}$$

The extent of the bell shape in a normal distribution depends on the standard deviation. Key properties of the normal distribution are that we can calculate the proportion of the observations that will lie between any two values of the variable, as long as we know the mean and standard deviation.

If observations follow a normal distribution, the standard deviation is a useful measure of the spread of these observations (**Figure 21**).

- A range covered by 1 SD above the mean and 1 SD below the mean includes 68% of the observations (ie the area under the curve).
- A range of 2 SDs (1.96) above and below the mean includes 95% of the observations.
- A range of 3 SDs (2.58) above and below the mean includes 99.7% of the observations.

The larger the standard deviation, the greater the spread of observations around the mean.

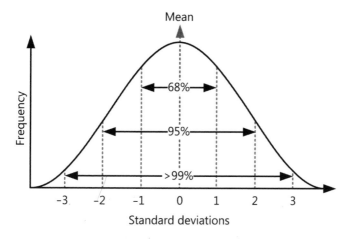

Figure 21 A normal distribution showing 1, 2 and 3 standard deviations

z score: Converts the value of an observation into the number of standard deviations that observation lies from the mean of the distribution. A z score is calculated by subtracting the mean from the observation and dividing the difference by the standard deviation. It is a dimensionless quantity. For example, a z score of 1.2 means the difference between the data point and mean value is +1.2 times the size of the standard deviation of the population. A negative z score indicates that the value of the data point is less than the mean. It is possible to calculate the probability of getting a value with a certain z score.

Coefficient of variation: Used to compare studies using different units which makes direct comparisons difficult. It is a measure of spread that is independent of the unit of measurement. The coefficient of variation is the ratio of the standard deviation and the mean and is expressed as a percentage.

$$\text{coefficient of variation} = \frac{\text{standard deviation}}{\text{mean}} \times 100$$

Standard normal distribution: A special case of the normal distribution in which the mean is zero, the variance (and standard deviation) is 1 and the area under the curve is equal to 1. Normal distributions can be converted to standard normal distributions. This transformation enables comparisons of distributions that have different means by showing them on the same scale.

Effect size: The effect size is used to compare the results of studies which used different outcome measures. It is calculated for each study by the following equation:

$$\text{effect size} = \frac{(\text{mean in experimental group} - \text{mean in control group})}{\text{standard deviation of the control group or both groups}}$$

It is also known as the **standardised mean difference**. The larger the value of the effect size, the greater the impact of the intervention.

DESCRIBING NON-NORMALLY DISTRIBUTED DATA

Non-normally distributed data (median, range, interquartile range)

As shown in **Figure 22**, in non-normally distributed data the data values are distributed asymmetrically across the distribution.

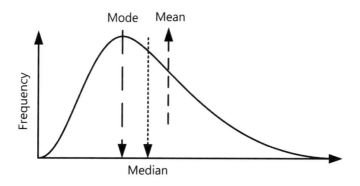

Figure 22 A non-normally distributed data set (positively skewed)

Median: From the Latin for 'middle', the median represents the middle value of ordered data observations. With an even number of data values, the median is the average of the two values that lie on either side of the middle (**Table 15**).

The advantage of the median estimation is that it is robust to outliers, meaning that it is not affected by aberrant points (unlike the mean). The main disadvantage of using the median is that it does not use all the data values in its determination.

Geometric mean: This is used when the distribution is positively skewed. Each value in the distribution is replaced by its logarithm to base e, resulting in a **log normal distribution**. The arithmetic mean is calculated on the new log-transformed scale and then transformed back using the exponential transformation to give a mean that is in the same units as the original data. If the distribution of the log data is approximately symmetrical, the geometric mean is similar to the median and less than the mean of the raw data.

Range: This is the difference between the lowest and highest values in the data set. It is useful for skewed data but it is not robust to aberrant values.

DATA SET	MEDIAN	RANGE
1, 2, 3, 3, 5	3	5 − 1 = 4
1, 2, 3, 3, 5, 7, 8, 10	(3+5 / 2) = 4	10 − 1 = 9

Table 15 Example calculations of median and range

Interquartile range: This is a 'mini' range because it focuses on the spread of the middle 50% of the data. It is usually reported alongside the median value of the data set.

The data are ranked in order and divided into four equal parts (irrespective of their values). The points at 25%, 50% and 75% of the distribution are identified. These are known as the quartiles and the median is the second quartile. The interquartile range is between the first and third quartiles (**Figure 23**).

Unlike the range, the interquartile range is not influenced by outliers and is relatively easy to calculate. However, the interquartile range does not incorporate all the presented values.

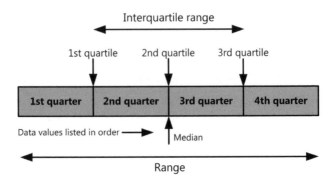

Figure 23 Comparing the range and the interquartile range

If the number of data values is not divisible by 4, first identify the median value and then calculate the first and third quartiles by the middle values between the median and the end of the ranges.

Percentiles or centiles: The data set is divided into 100 equal parts. These are sometimes used to define the normal ranges for clinical measures:
- 10% of the values lie below the 10th percentile
- 20% of the values lie below the 20th percentile
- 50% of the values lie below the 50th percentile (median)

Measures of shape

Skewness might be obvious when the data are presented on a histogram or scatter diagram.

The **coefficient of skewness** is a measure of symmetry.

The **coefficient of kurtosis** measures the peakedness of a distribution.

- **Positively skewed distribution:** The distribution has an extended tail to the right and has a positive coefficient of skewness. The mean is larger than the median, which is larger than the mode.

- **Negatively skewed distribution:** The distribution has an extended tail to the left and has a negative coefficient of skewness. The mean is smaller than the median, which is smaller than the mode.

- **Symmetrical distribution:** This has a coefficient of skewness of zero.

Transforming data

Even for data that are not distributed normally, the data are often transformed into a distribution to allow statistical tests to be used. For example, skewed data can be transformed into a normal distribution and curved relationships can be made linear. Examples of transformations are the use of logarithms, reciprocals and square roots of the data values.

Self-assessment exercise 11

1. In this data set: 1, 2, 2, 3, 3, 3, 4, 4, 5
    a. What is the mode?
    b. What is the frequency?
    c. What is the median?
    d. What is the range?
    e. What is the mean?

2. In this data set: 5, 10, 15, 20, 100
    a. What is the median?
    b. What is the range?
    c. What is the mean?
    d. Which describes the central tendency of this data set better – the median or the mean?

3. In this data set: 5, 10, 15, 20, 25, 30, 35, 40, 45, 50, 60, 70
    a. What is the median?
    b. What is the range?
    c. What is the interquartile range?

4. In this data set: 3, 13, 44, 45, 51, 56, 66, 75, 91, 102
    a. What is the mean?
    b. What is the standard deviation?
    c. What is the range in which 95% of observations will lie?

To generalise the result from a random sample to the target population, two concepts need to be understood:

- Standard error
- Confidence intervals

Standard error of the mean (SE)

Imagine that an experiment is set up to measure the mean height of the population. A random sample of the population will be selected to take part in the study. The results from the sample will be generalised to the population.

If the study is repeated with a new random sample, the mean height from this new sample might not be the same as that from the first random sample. Indeed, repeating the study several times might produce a series of different mean heights. This is shown in **Table 16**.

	MEAN HEIGHT	STANDARD DEVIATION
Sample 1	1.65	0.12
Sample 2	1.58	0.23
Sample 3	1.63	0.19
Sample 4	1.88	0.22
Sample 5	1.59	0.18
Sample 6	1.44	0.20
Sample 7	1.63	0.05
Sample 8	1.49	0.14

Table 16 Mean heights (in metres) and standard deviations from different samples

If these sample means are themselves plotted on a graph, the sampling distribution of the mean will follow a normal distribution (**Figure 24**). The mean of all the sample means is the same as the population mean. The standard deviation of the sample means has its own name, the **standard error of the mean**, often shortened to **standard error** and abbreviated to SE.

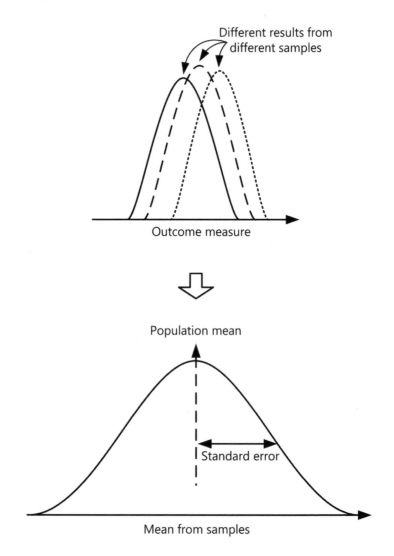

Figure 24 Population mean and standard error

$$\text{standard error of a sample of size } n = \frac{\text{standard deviation}}{\sqrt{n}}$$

n = number of observations in the sample

The standard error of the mean is a measure of the precision of the sample mean as an estimate of the population mean. The more observations you have, the smaller the standard error will be – that is, the more likely it is that the sample mean ($\bar{x}$) reflects the true mean value (μ) of a parameter in the general population. The standard error can be used to assess the sampling error by indicating how close a sample mean is to the population mean it is estimating.

Confidence intervals (CI)

Imagine that we want to know the mean height of 500 pupils attending a school.

- If all 500 pupils are in our sample, we are 100% confident that we will calculate the correct mean height from all the height measurements we take.

- If our sample is 499 pupils, we are still very confident that the mean height we calculate from our sample will be very similar to the mean height of the target population. The mean height for all 500 pupils might be a bit higher or a bit lower, but the difference, if it exists, will be very small indeed.

- If our sample is 400 pupils, we are slightly less confident that the mean value we calculate lies close to the real mean value for all the pupils. If we had to guess where the real value lies, we would quote a small range either side of the value we have calculated.

- If our sample is only 50 pupils, we would be even less confident in our result. Even if the result is correct, we don't know it is, so we are less confident. The range in which we think the true value lies will be wider.

Confidence intervals measure the uncertainty in measurements. They can be described as a range of values which, when quoted in relation to an estimate from a sample, express the degree of uncertainty around that estimate.

The width of the confidence interval indicates the **precision** of the estimate. The 95% confidence interval is routinely quoted; it is the range within which we can be 95% confident that the true value for the population lies. For example, for a mean height of 1.25 m with a 95% confidence interval of 1.1 m and 1.4 m, we are 95% confident that the true mean height value lies between 1.1 m and 1.4 m.

We can make a wide estimate with a high degree of confidence or a more precise estimate with a lower degree of confidence. The larger the sample, the less variable the observations are, and the more likely the results are to be true – that is, the narrower the confidence interval and the more confidence one can have in making inferences about the population parameters.

95% confidence interval for a population mean
= mean ± (1.96 × standard error)

- When quoted alongside a difference between two groups (eg mean difference), a confidence interval that includes 0 is statistically non-significant.

- When quoted alongside a ratio (eg relative risk, odds ratio), a confidence interval that includes 1 is statistically non-significant.

Confidence intervals involving ratios, such as relative risk or odds ratios, are usually asymmetrical and do not use the plus or minus type formula. Asymmetrical confidence intervals can be transformed into symmetrical confidence intervals if a log scale is used instead.

Self-assessment exercise 12

1. In this data set: 10, 12, 15, 17, 18, 19, 21
   a. What is the mean?
   b. What is the median?
   c. What is the standard deviation?
   d. What is the standard error?

2. In this data set: 10, 12, 15, 17, 18, 19, 91
   a. What is the mean?
   b. What is the median?
   c. What is the standard deviation?
   d. What is the standard error?

COMPARING SAMPLES –
THE NULL HYPOTHESIS

The results from two or more groups are often being compared in research. The researcher is interested in finding out if there are any differences between the groups because this could highlight an important role for an exposure, investigation or treatment.

To complicate matters, by convention this task is turned on its head, with the researcher assuming that any differences seen are due to chance. The researcher then calculates how likely it is that such differences are indeed due to chance, hoping to show that it is in fact very unlikely.

Step one – the null hypothesis

The **null hypothesis** states that any difference observed in the results of two or more groups is due to chance. The null hypothesis is rarely stated in clinical papers and should not be confused with the primary hypothesis. The importance of the null hypothesis lies in the fact that it underpins the statistical tests.

For example, the initial research question might be, 'Does a relationship exist between cannabis smoking and the development of schizophrenia?' The researcher might set up a case–control study to look at past cannabis smoking in a group of schizophrenic patients and matched controls. If there are differences in exposure to cannabis smoking between the two groups, the researcher dismisses this difference in terms of the null hypothesis, ie that 'no relationship exists between cannabis use and schizophrenia'. The researcher then uses statistical tests to calculate the probability that the difference in cannabis smoking prevalence is indeed due to chance and to decide whether this probability is large enough to accept, in which case the null hypothesis stands true.

If the results are unlikely to be explained by chance alone, the null hypothesis is rejected and the **alternative hypothesis**, which states that there is a difference that is not due to chance, is accepted.

Step two – calculating probabilities

Probability is the likelihood of any event occurring as a proportion of the total number of possibilities. The probability of an event varies between 0.0 (never happens) to 1.0 (certain to happen).

Probability in clinical papers is often expressed as the **'P value'**. P values express the probability of getting the observed results given a true null hypothesis. P values are calculated using statistical methods.

As the P value becomes smaller, the difference between the observed results becomes less and less compatible with the null hypothesis. Eventually the P value is so small that the study data can no longer be accepted as supporting the null hypothesis. The P value at which this decision is taken is called the significance level.

By convention, a P value of less than 0.05 is the accepted threshold for **statistical significance** – that is, the null hypothesis can be rejected. $P < 0.05$ means that the probability of obtaining a given result by chance is less than 1 in 20. The text in the paper might express this as, 'The results are significant at the 5% level.'

P values greater than 0.05 are statistically non-significant – that is, the null hypothesis is accepted.

This is summarised in **Table 17**. The roles of probability in rejecting the null hypothesis is explained in another way in **Table 18**. P values can be calculated using several statistical techniques.

$P < 0.05$	$P \geq 0.05$
Less than 1 in 20	Greater than 1 in 20
Results statistically significant	Results statistically non-significant
Null hypothesis is rejected	Null hypothesis is accepted
Evidence of association between variable and outcome	Association between variable and outcome not proved

Table 17 Understanding P values and significance

EVENT	WHAT OTHER PEOPLE SAY	WHAT A RESEARCHER SAYS
Week 1 Dr Cash wins £5 million on the National Lottery.	He is as likely as anyone else to win the lottery. His win was due to chance.	Null hypothesis: Dr Cash is no more likely to win the lottery than anyone else. The null hypothesis holds true.
Week 2 Dr Cash wins the National Lottery again.	He is as likely to win as anyone else, even though he won it last week too. He's just incredibly lucky.	Null hypothesis: Dr Cash is no more likely to win the lottery than anyone else. The probability of his winning twice in 2 weeks is even more unlikely but it can happen. The null hypothesis holds true.
Week 3 Dr Cash wins the National Lottery for the third week in a row.	We suspect Dr Cash has not won the lottery three times simply by chance. There is something else going on here to explain these events.	The null hypothesis is **rejected** – the association between Dr Cash and the three consecutive lottery wins is not due simply to chance. The probability of this happening is so small that it is not acceptable.

Table 18 The role of probability in rejecting the null hypothesis

Step 3 – consider type 1 and type 2 errors

Type 1 errors

The possibility of a type 1 error should be considered with every significant finding.

A type 1 error occurs when the null hypothesis is rejected when it is true. A **false-positive** result has been recorded because a difference is found between groups when no such difference exists. Type 1 errors are usually attributable to bias, confounding or multiple hypothesis testing. The methodology of the study must be scrutinised for these problems.

If a difference is seen between two groups, significance testing must take place to avoid making a type 1 error. P values should be quoted alongside the results. $P = 0.05$ is used as the level of risk we are prepared to take that we will make a type 1 error. The probability of making a type 1 error is equal to P and expressed as α. For example $\alpha = 0.05$ means that there is only a 5% chance of erroneously rejecting the null hypothesis.

Type 2 errors

The possibility of a type 2 error should be considered with every non-significant finding.

A type 2 error occurs when the null hypothesis is accepted when it is in fact false. The study has returned a **false-negative** result after failing to uncover a difference between the groups that actually exists. This usually happens because the sample size is not large enough and/or the measurement variance is too large.

Type 2 errors can be avoided at the design stage of the study by power calculations that give an indication of how many subjects are required in the trial to minimise the risk of making a type 2 error. The probability of making a type 2 error is expressed as β.

Figure 25 and **Table 19** summarise the discussion so far.

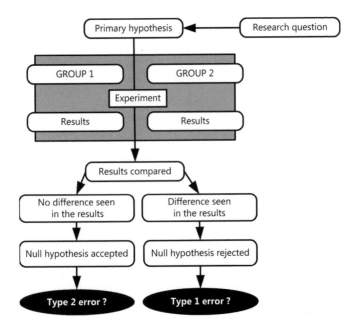

Figure 25 The null hypothesis, type 1 error and type 2 error

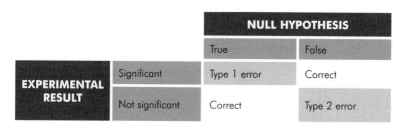

		NULL HYPOTHESIS	
		True	False
EXPERIMENTAL RESULT	Significant	Type 1 error	Correct
	Not significant	Correct	Type 2 error

Table 19 Type 1 and 2 errors

Sample size and power

The **sample size** for a study is not simply chosen at random. Ideally, a clinical trial should be large enough to reliably detect the smallest possible difference in the outcome measure, with treatment, that is considered clinically worthwhile.

The **power** of a study is its ability to detect the smallest clinically significant difference in outcome between the control arm and the intervention arm, if such a difference exits. This is defined as the probability that a type 2 error will not be made in that study.

Power calculations are made to ensure that the study is large enough to have a high chance of detecting a statistically significant result if one truly exists. As a general rule, the larger the sample size of a study, the more power the study is said to have.

It is not uncommon for studies to be underpowered, failing to detect even large treatment effects because of an inadequate sample size. A calculation should be performed at the start of a study to determine the degree of power chosen for that study. For example, a power of 0.8 means there is an 80% probability of finding a significant difference with a given sample size, if a real difference truly does exist, having excluded the role of chance. **A power of 0.8 is generally accepted as being adequate in most research studies.** A study power set at 80% accepts a likelihood of 1 in 5 (ie 20%) of missing such a real difference.

The probability of rejecting the null hypothesis when a true difference exists is represented as $1 - \beta$. Typically, β is arbitrarily set at 0.2, meaning that a study has 80% power (0.8 of a chance) to detect a specified degree of difference at a specified degree of significance.

Power calculations can also be used to calculate the minimum effect size that is likely to be detected in a study using a given sample size and power.

The key to avoiding type 2 errors is to power the study adequately. In new clinical fields, pilot studies might be carried out to estimate the difference in outcomes between experimental and control groups in order to inform a power calculation. Sometimes studies in progress are double-checked by performing an interim analysis.

A cautious researcher may recruit more subjects than is absolutely required by a power calculation, to maintain adequate numbers in the trial even if some subjects drop out. A power calculation can also be used to discourage researchers from recruiting too many subjects, however, bearing in mind that the excess subjects might be allocated to an inferior or ineffective intervention arm.

The **determinants of power** are:

- The **α level** that is set. Power is increased with larger α levels because a type 1 error is more likely.
- The **sample size**. Power is increased with larger sample sizes.
- The **variability of the outcome measure**, as defined by its standard deviation. Power is increased as the variability decreases.
- The **minimum clinically significant difference**. Power is increased with larger clinically significant differences. This difference can be given as a difference in means or proportions. When it is expressed as a multiple of the standard deviations of the observations it is called the **standardised difference**.

One-tailed versus two-tailed tests

The **alternative hypothesis** is the proposed experimental hypothesis that runs opposite to the null hypothesis. The null hypothesis states that there is no difference between two or more groups. If the null hypothesis is not true, the alternative hypothesis must be true.

Depending on the alternative hypothesis, there might be a choice between one-tailed and two-tailed significance tests.

A **two-tailed test** exists if the alternative hypothesis does not offer a direction for the difference between the groups. One group could do better or worse than the other group. It allows for either eventuality and is recommended as we are rarely certain, in advance, of the direction of any difference, if one exists.

If the alternative hypothesis does specify a direction, the result is a **one-tailed test**. This could be the case, for example, when comparing a new intervention with a placebo, where we would not expect the placebo group to do better. With a one-tailed test, the null hypothesis is modified slightly to state that there is no difference between the groups or that the placebo group does better. One-tailed tests are not used often but, when they are, the direction of difference should be specified in advance. The opposite direction is disregarded.

Bonferroni correction

Some research studies include a large number of significance tests. It is expected that 5% of significance tests (1 out of 20) would be significant purely due to chance. The more tests that are carried out, the more likely it is that a type 1 error will be made.

The **Bonferroni correction** safeguards against multiple tests of statistical significance on the same data which might falsely give the appearance of significance. It does this by adjusting the statistical significance level for the number of tests that have been performed on the data. A Bonferroni correction makes it harder to achieve a significant result.

If the Bonferroni correction is excessive, it will increase the risk of making a type 2 error.

Clinical significance

Statistical significance as shown by P values is not the same as **clinical significance**. Statistical significance judges whether treatment effects are explicable as chance findings. Clinical significance assesses whether treatment effects are worthwhile in real life. Small improvements that are statistically significant might not result in any meaningful improvement clinically, for example.

Confidence intervals and significance

A significance result can be deduced from comparing the confidence intervals associated with the summary statistics from two groups. A confidence interval is normally the range of values around a summary statistic in which we are 95% sure the population summary statistic lies.

- When comparing two groups, if the confidence intervals do not overlap this is equivalent to a significant result.

- If the confidence intervals overlap but one summary statistic is not within the confidence interval of the other, the result might be significant.

- If the confidence intervals overlap and the summary statistics are within the confidence interval of the other, the result is not significant.

Which is better – a confidence interval or a P value? Both can indicate statistical significance. The P value provides a measure of the strength of an association. The confidence interval indicates the magnitude of an effect and likely clinical implications because it indicates a range of possible values for the true effect in the target population.

Larger studies will in general result in narrower confidence intervals and smaller P values, and this should be taken into account when interpreting the results from statistical analyses.

Self-assessment exercise 13

How would you write the following clinical questions in terms of the null hypothesis?

1.   Do patients have problems when they stop paroxetine suddenly?

2.   Is atorvastatin more effective than simvastatin at lowering cholesterol levels?

Samples are compared using a variety of statistical tests. Not all statistical tests can be used with all data sets. The determining factors are the number of samples we are comparing, the type of data in the samples, the distribution of the samples and whether the data are paired or unpaired.

Unpaired data refers to data from two groups which have different members. Here the selection of the individuals for one group must not be influenced by or related to the selection of the other group. **Paired data** refers to data from the same individuals at different time points.

Table 20 summarises the statistical tests that can be used when the types of data collected from the study are the same. As most biological variables are normally distributed, the t test is one of the most popular statistical tests for comparing two sets of data.

	CATEGORICAL DATA	NON-NORMAL DATA	NORMAL DATA
One sample compared with a hypothetical sample	Chi-squared test Fisher's exact test (small sample)	Sign test Wilcoxon's signed rank test	One-sample t test
Comparing two groups of data	Chi-squared test (unpaired) Fisher's exact test (unpaired, small sample) McNemar's test (paired)	Mann–Whitney U test (unpaired) (equivalent to the Wilcoxon's rank sum test) Wilcoxon's matched pairs test (paired)	t test (paired or unpaired)
Comparing more than two groups of data	Chi-squared test (unpaired) McNemar's test (paired)	Kruskal–Wallis ANOVA test (unpaired) Friedman's test (paired)	One-way ANOVA for unpaired groups Repeated-measures ANOVA for paired groups

Table 20 Summary of statistical tests used for comparing samples, ANOVA, analysis of variance

Categorical data

Categorical statistical tests involve the use of **contingency tables**, also known as **2 × 2 tables** (**Table 21**). Remember that 'outcome event yes' always refers to the worst outcome possible, such as death.

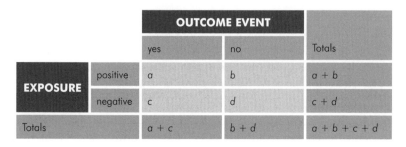

		OUTCOME EVENT		
		yes	no	Totals
EXPOSURE	positive	a	b	a + b
	negative	c	d	c + d
Totals		a + c	b + d	a + b + c + d

Table 21 The format of a 2 × table

The statistical tests used with categorical data are the chi-squared (χ^2) test (unpaired data) and McNemar's test (paired binary data).

For small-sized samples (fewer than five observations in any cell), Fisher's exact test can be used (**Figure 26**). Alternatively, the **Yates continuity correction** can be used to make the chi-squared statistic have better agreement with Fisher's exact test when the sample size is small.

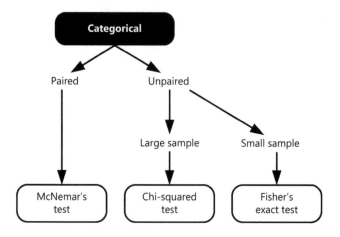

Figure 26 The statistical tests used with categorical data

Degrees of freedom: This is an estimate of the number of independent categories in a particular statistical test or experiment. Dependent categories can be calculated from the independent categories. In the case of a 2 × 2 contingency table, it is the number of ways in which the results in the table can vary, given the column and row totals. A 2 × 2 table has two columns and two rows. If the result in one of the row cells is changed, the result in the other row cell can be calculated. Similarly, if the result in one of the column cells is changed, the result in the other column cell can be calculated. Degrees of freedom is therefore:

$$(\text{number of rows} - 1) \times (\text{number of columns} - 1)$$

Continuous data

Non-parametric tests, also referred to as 'distribution-free statistics', are used for analysis of non-normally distributed data (**Table 22**). The most commonly used tests for two independent groups are the Mann–Whitney U test (unpaired data) and Wilcoxon's matched pairs test (for paired data). The most commonly used tests for two or more groups are the Kruskal–Wallis analysis of variance (ANOVA) (for unpaired data) and Friedman's test (paired data) (**Figure 27**).

The sign test is the simplest of all the non-parametric methods. It is used to compare a single sample with some hypothesised value and it is therefore useful in those situations in which the one-sample t test or paired t test might traditionally be applied.

NON-NORMALLY DISTRIBUTED DATA		
Statistical test	**Data**	**Explanation**
Sign test Wilcoxon's signed rank test	One sample data	The median of the sample is compared with a hypothetical mean
Mann–Whitney U test (equivalent to Wilcoxon's rank sum test)	Two unpaired samples	The median of one sample is compared with the median of another sample
Wilcoxon's matched-pairs test	Two paired samples	The median of one sample is compared with the median of another sample
Kruskal–Wallis ANOVA test	Three or more samples of unpaired data	The medians of samples from three or more groups are compared
Friedman's test	Three or more samples of paired data	The medians of samples from three or more groups are compared

Table 22 Statistical tests and non-normally distributed data

Non-normally distributed data can either be mathematically transformed into a normal-like distribution by taking powers, reciprocals or logarithms of data values or, alternatively, statistical tests can be used that don't have the assumption of normality.

Parametric tests are used for data that are normally distributed (**Table 23**). The Z test is essentially the same as the t test and can be used with unpaired data from larger sample sizes ($n>30$).

NORMALLY DISTRIBUTED DATA		
Statistical test	**Data**	**Explanation**
One-sample *t* test	One sample data	The mean of the sample is compared with a hypothetical mean
t test	Two unpaired samples	The mean of one sample is compared with the mean of another sample
Paired *t* test	Two paired samples	The mean of one sample is compared with the mean of another sample
Analysis of variance	Three or more samples of unpaired or paired data	The means of samples from three or more groups are compared

Table 23 Statistical tests and normally distributed data

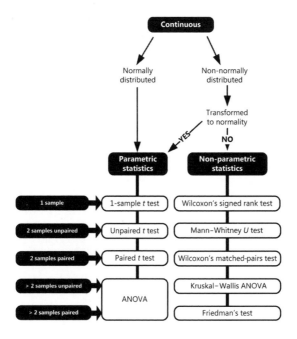

Figure 27 The statistical tests used with continuous data

Additional statistical analyses

The rest of this chapter, including the next three tables (**Tables 24–26**) summarises information on advanced statistical analysis (CI = confidence interval; IQR = interquartile range; OR = odds ratio; RR = relative risk). This information is provided for reference only and would not be needed in everyday critical appraisal work.

Statistics used for different scales

	NOMINAL	ORDINAL	INTERVAL	RATIO
Descriptive statistics	Mode	Median	Mean Standard deviation	All
Analytical statistics	Chi-squared test	Percentile	Correlation Regression ANOVA	All

Table 24 Statistics used for different scales

Statistics used when there is only one outcome variable

		NUMBER OF MEASUREMENTS PER SUBJECT		
		One	Two	Three or more
OUTCOME VARIABLE	Categorical Binary	Incidence/ prevalence and 95% CI	Kappa McNemar's test	—
	Continuous	Mean, standard deviation and 95% CI Median and IQR One-sample *t* test	Intraclass correlation coefficient Mean difference and 95% CI Measurement error Paired *t* test	Repeated-measures analysis of variance

Table 25 Statistics used when there is only one outcome variable

Statistics used when there is one dependent and one independent variable

		INDEPENDENT VARIABLE	
		CATEGORICAL	**CONTINUOUS**
DEPENDENT VARIABLE (OUTCOME)	**CATEGORICAL**	**Both variables binary:** Chi-squared test Likelihood ratio Logistic regression OR / RR Sensitivity or specificity	**Categorical variable is binary:** Survival analysis
		One or more of the variables has more than two levels: Kendall's correlation	**Categorical variable is multilevel and ordered:** Spearman's correlation coefficient
	CONTINUOUS	**Categorical variable binary:** Independent samples *t* test Mean difference and 95% CI	Pearson's correlation Regression
		Categorical variable has 3 or more categories: ANOVA	

Table 26 Statistics used when there is one dependent and one independent variable

Analysis of variance (ANOVA)

ANOVA is used to compare the means of three or more groups of continuous or interval scores.

- **A one-way ANOVA** is used when the effect of only one categorical variable (explanatory variable) on a single continuous variable (outcome) is assessed, eg the effect of ethnicity on cholesterol level.

- **A factorial ANOVA / two-way ANOVA** is used when the effects of two or more categorical variables on a single continuous variable are assessed, eg the effect of ethnicity and socioeconomic status on height.

- In **repeated-measures ANOVA** the same measure is used on more than one occasion in the same group of patients and it tests the equality of means.

ANOVA also has some multivariate extensions:

- **ANCOVA** (analysis of covariance): This is used when the effects of one or more of the categorical explanatory variables on a single continuous outcome variable are explored after adjusting for one or more continuous variables. These are called 'covariates'. An example is the effects of gender and ethnicity on cholesterol level after adjusting for weight.

- **MANOVA** (multiple analysis of variance): This is used with multiple dependent variables and is useful for multiple hypothesis testing.

- **MANCOVA** (multiple analysis of covariance): This is used with multiple dependent and independent variables.

A researcher may pit a new drug against a placebo preparation to illustrate the new drug's efficacy in the management of a condition. However, a placebo-controlled trial does not give clinicians the information they want if there is already a treatment available for the condition. In that situation a trial comparing a new drug to the standard drug is more useful.

A researcher can of course set up a trial to assess whether a new drug is better than the standard drug. In such **superiority trials** significance testing is used to determine if there is a difference between the treatments. Superiority studies require large numbers of subjects to ensure adequate power and to minimise type 2 errors because less difference is expected when a new treatment is compared with a standard treatment instead of with a placebo.

Equivalence
In an **equivalence study** the researcher attempts to show equivalence between drugs. It is difficult to show exact equivalence so the trial is designed to demonstrate that any difference in outcome between the two drugs lies within a specified range called the 'equivalence margin' or 'delta'. Delta should represent the smallest clinically acceptable difference. Equivalence can be assumed if the confidence interval around the observed difference in effect between the two drugs lies entirely within delta[1]. If the equivalence margin is too wide, the risk of getting a false–positive result increases (the two drugs are wrongly accepted as equivalent).

Non-inferiority
In a **non-inferiority study** the researcher assesses whether a new drug is no worse within a specified margin than the standard drug. If the confidence interval for the difference between the two drugs is not more negative than a pre-specified amount, called the non-inferiority margin or delta, then non-inferiority can be assumed[1]. A non-inferiority study is a one-sided version of an equivalence study. Inferiority trails should be avoided in situations where any

1   Piaggio G, Elbourne DR, Altman DG, Pocock SJ, Evans SJ. Reporting of noninferiority and equivalence randomized trials: An extension of the CONSORT statement. *JAMA* 2006, 295, 1152–60.

inferiority is unacceptable, for example where the treatment is used to avoid a seriously undesirable outcome such as death.

What is the purpose of non-inferiority trials? The answer is that pharmaceutical companies might not need to show that their new drug is better than the standard drug in order to gain market share. For example, if a drug can be shown to be non-inferior and has advantages such as being cheaper or causing fewer adverse effects, the new drug is likely to be prescribed by clinicians. Non-inferiority trials usually require smaller sample sizes and are cheaper and quicker to run than superiority or equivalence trials. Once non-inferiority has been established, further statistical tests can be performed on the data to test for superiority.

Selecting interventions based on class effect

Grouping drugs together depends on the drugs having similar characteristics, which may include chemical structure, pharmacokinetics and pharmacodynamics. A **class effect** exists if the drugs grouped together have similar therapeutic effects and similar adverse effects.

Choosing a drug which belongs to a group and which shares a class effect is relatively straightforward, as usually the cheapest option is selected.

So far, we have described the data from a single sample, inferred population data from data samples and compared samples using the null hypothesis. Sometimes it is necessary to establish the nature of the relationship between two or more variables to see if they are associated.

Multivariate statistics enable us to examine the relationships between several variables and make predictions about the data set. There are several methods, depending on the number of variables being examined.

Continuous data can be analysed using correlation and regression techniques.

Correlation

Correlation assesses the **strength** of the relationship between two quantitative variables (**Figure 28**). It examines whether a linear association exists between two variables, X and Y. X is usually the independent variable and Y is usually the dependent variable.

- A **positive correlation** means that Y increases linearly as X increases.

- A **negative correlation** means that Y decreases linearly as X increases.

- **Zero correlation** reflects a complete non-association between the compared variables.

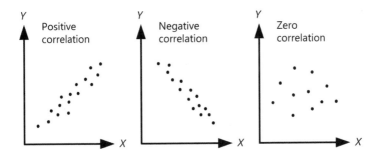

Figure 28 Scatter graphs illustrating three types of correlation

Correlation coefficient

The relationship on a scatter graph can be quantified by the correlation coefficient (r):

- If r is positive the variables are directly related. As one variable increases, so does the other.
- If r is negative the variables are inversely related. As one variable increases, the other decreases.
- r has no units.
- The value of r varies from -1 to $+1$:
  - if $r = 0$ there is no correlation
  - the closer r is to 0, the weaker the correlation
  - if $r = -1$ or $r = +1$ there is perfect correlation (all the points fall on a line)
  - the closer r is to -1 or $+1$, the stronger the correlation
  - r is regarded as strong if $r < -0.5$ or $r > 0.5$
  - r is not the gradient of the line – the value of r reflects both the direction of any relationship and how tight that relationship is

Correlation coefficients are usually presented with P values. The null hypothesis states that there is no correlation. The P value is dependent on the strength of the correlation but also the sample size, so a small correlation coefficient can be statistically significant if the sample size is large and vice versa, making interpretation more difficult.

The square of the correlation coefficient (**r^2**) is the **coefficient of determination**, an estimate of the percentage variation in one variable that is explained by the other variable. This is useful when interpreting clinical relevance. For example, the correlation between exam revision and exam results was found to be 0.8, indicating the importance of revision in exam results. In this case $r^2 = 0.8 \times 0.8 = 0.64$. This means that 64% of the variation in exam results was accounted for by the amount of revision done. Other factors, such as inborn intelligence, account for the rest of the variation in exam results.

Correlation coefficients describe **associations**, that two or more variables vary in a related way. Correlation coefficients do not describe causal relationships.

Even when there is a strong correlation between X and Y, explanations can include any of the following:

- This correlation is a chance finding.
- X partly determines the value of Y.
- Y partly determines the value of X.
- The changes in X and Y are explained by a confounding variable.

There are different types of correlation coefficients. The correlation coefficient used to describe the relationship between two variables depends on the type of data being compared.

Pearson's correlation coefficient (r): This parametric statistic measures the linear association between two variables, giving an indication as to whether the paired values lie on a straight line. At least one of the variables must be normally distributed and the relationship is linear.

Spearman's rank correlation (rho, ρ) and Kendall's correlation coefficient (tau, τ): These are non-parametric measures of correlation based on ranks. Kendall's correlation coefficient is based on the probability that the rank orders are different, whereas Spearman's rank correlation coefficient is based on the degree of variability in rank order of one variable accounted for by the other. Assumptions are that the variables can be ranked and that the relationship between the variables either increases or decreases.

Regression

Whereas correlation quantifies the strength of the linear relationship between a pair of variables, regression expresses the relationship between two or more variables in the form of an equation.

Regression determines the nature of the relationship between two or more variables. It involves estimating the best straight line to summarise the association.

The relationship between variables can be represented by the regression line on a scatter graph. The regression line is constructed using a regression equation. The regression equation has predictive value but it does not prove causality.

Simple linear regression (univariate regression)

Simple linear regression is concerned with describing the linear relationship between a dependent (outcome) variable, Y, and single explanatory (independent or predictor) variable, X. Standard errors can be estimated and confidence intervals can be determined.

Where there is one independent variable, the equation of the best fit for the regression line is:

$Y = a + bX$

Y = the value of the dependent variable

a = intercept of the regression line on the Y axis, ie the value of Y when $X = 0$

b = regression coefficient (slope or gradient of the regression line), describing the strength of the relationship

X = the value of the independent variable

For a given value of X, a corresponding value of Y can be predicted (see **Figure 29**). The predicted values should be presented with their 95% confidence intervals to indicate the precision with which they have been estimated.

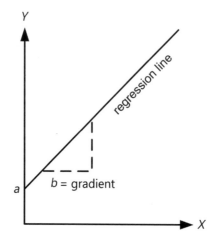

Figure 29 Simple linear regression

Method of least squares

This method determines which is the best of several tentative lines drawn on a scatter plot. At each attempt, the vertical distance(s) of each data observation from the tentative line is measured and squared. All squared distances are added together to produce a 'sum of squared distances' measure for that tentative line. The eventual linear regression line is determined by finding the line that results in the least 'sum of squared distances'.

Multiple linear regression (multivariable regression)

A regression model in which the dependent outcome variable is predicted from two or more independent variables is called 'multiple linear regression'. The independent variables can be continuous or categorical.

A measure of association is calculated taking a number of variables into account simultaneously:

$$Y = a + b_1X_1 + b_2X_2 + ...$$

$a = Y$ when all the independent variables are zero

$b_1, b_2, ...$ = partial regression coefficients for each independent variable

The partial regression coefficients are calculated by the **least squares method**. This is usually presented along with a 95% confidence interval and a P value. If $P < 0.05$ or the confidence interval does not contain zero, then the independent variable has a significant influence on the dependent variable.

Multiple linear regression is used to assess what effect different variables might have on the study outcome. It is also used to assess the effects of possible confounding factors that may be present in the study.

Logistic regression

Linear and multiple regression assume that the dependent variable is continuous. Logistic regression is used when we have a binary outcome of interest. It has a theoretical binomial distribution.

Regression models cannot be fitted directly to binary variables. Instead, the outcome measure is based on the probabilities of each category occurring, eg failure/success; presence/absence of a disease.

Proportional Cox regression

This is also known as the 'proportional hazards regression' and can be used to determine the influence of variables on survival or on other time-related events. The outcome measure used is not actual survival time. Instead, the concept of hazard rate is used. See also page 178.

Factor analysis

This is a statistical approach that can be used to analyse inter-relationships among a large number of variables and can be used to explain these variables in terms of their common underlying factors.

Cluster analysis

This is a multivariate analysis technique that tries to organise information about variables so that relatively homogeneous groups (clusters) can be formed.

SYSTEMATIC REVIEWS AND META-ANALYSES

So far, we have been critically appraising individual studies. However, a literature search often reveals many studies with similar aims and hypotheses. Examining one study in isolation can mean that we miss out on findings discovered by other researchers. Ideally, all the studies around one subject area should be collated.

Reviews of articles provide a useful summary of the literature in a particular field. The main flaw with many of these reviews is that they are based on a selection of papers collected in a non-systematic way, so that important research might have been missed.

Systematic review

A systematic review attempts to access and review systematically all of the pertinent articles in the field. A systematic review should effectively explain the research question, the search strategy and the designs of the studies that were selected. The results of these studies are then pooled. The evidence drawn from systematic reviews can therefore be very powerful and valuable. The overall conclusions are more accurate and reliable than those of individual studies. Systematic reviews are the gold-standard source of research evidence in the hierarchy of research evidence.

There are four key components to systematic reviews (**Table 27**).

Research question	Prespecification of study types Subjects, inclusion criteria, exclusion criteria Interventions, exposures Outcomes Statistical methods
Search strategy	Reproducible Comprehensive Unbiased
Quality assessment	Standardised proforma Study methodology details Assessment of study quality
Interpretation of the data	Fixed or random effects models Publication bias for small negative studies Heterogeneity

Table 27 Components of systematic reviews

Research question

As with all research, a systematic review should begin with a focused clinical question. The study types, outcomes of interest, inclusion criteria and exclusion criteria should be clearly stated.

Search strategy

A systematic review is only as good as the search strategy employed to find evidence. To avoid accusations of bias, the search should transcend geographical, language, cultural, academic and political barriers.

- A good systematic review will give a comprehensive account of the search strategy. This usually starts with a search of electronic databases, such as MEDLINE and EMBASE, and trial registers. Search terms include types of studies, exposures and outcomes. To aid transparency, the search terms and Boolean operators ('and', 'or', 'not') can be listed, together with the number of search results returned. This will enable other researchers to assess the thoroughness of the search strategy and allow the search to be repeated.

- Bibliographies of the identified articles can be scanned. Although this hand-searching technique is labour-intensive, links to more articles might be uncovered. Hand-searching can be extended to other sources of information, including grey literature. One advantage of manually searching the content lists of recent journals is that articles not yet included in medical databases might be found.

- Citation searching involves searching for articles that cite studies that have already been identified, with the expectation that such articles will be closely related and therefore relevant to the systematic review.

- The researchers may contact recognised experts and organisations in the field to find out about any other ongoing, missed or unpublished evidence.

Quality assessment

The abstracts of all the identified articles are reviewed and the studies that are deemed suitable are selected for a full review. Each article is then examined to ensure that it meets eligibility requirements and quality thresholds. Essentially, every piece of research is critically appraised with a view to eliminating biased studies that could overestimate or underestimate the treatment effect size. Reasons should be given for excluding studies.

This process is normally carried out by more than one researcher. The level of agreement between the researchers might be given. Any disagreements about whether a study should be included in the review are dealt with using agreed procedures in order to reach a consensus.

Interpretation of the data

Comparing data from different studies involves identifying common units of measurement. Outcomes such as relative risks and odds ratios are usually straightforward to compare. Exposures can be more problematic. Different studies may describe different doses of risk factors or treatments, in which case the researchers should explain how such doses were standardised across the studies.

Meta-analysis

A meta-analysis is the quantitative assessment of a systematic review. It involves combining the results of independent studies. Meta-analyses are performed when more than one study has estimated the effect of an intervention and when there are no differences in participants, interventions and settings that are likely to affect the outcome significantly. It is also important that the outcome in the different trials has been measured in similar ways. A good meta-analysis is based on a systematic review of studies rather than a non-systematic review, which can introduce bias into the analysis.

The results from the studies are combined to produce an overall estimate of effect. As a meta-analysis combines the results of research done on many patients, the larger sample size means the overall estimate of effect is more likely to be accurate and with a smaller confidence interval. The analysis has increased power to detect small but significant effects, reducing the risk of making a type 2 error. A meta-analysis can provide conclusive evidence for or against an intervention, even when individual studies are inconclusive.

The key steps to remember for a meta-analysis are:

- Synthesis using statistical techniques to combine results of included studies
- Calculation of a pooled estimate of effect of an intervention together with its P value and confidence interval
- A check for variations between the studies (heterogeneity)
- A check for publication bias
- Review and interpretation of the findings

Forest plots

The results of a meta-analysis are presented as a forest plot (or blobbogram) of pooled results. **Figure 30** summarises the components of a forest plot.

The forest plot is a diagram with a list of studies on the vertical axis, often arranged in order of effect or chronologically, and the common outcome measure on the horizontal axis. The outcome measure can be odds or risk ratio, mean differences, event rates, etc. There is a vertical 'line of no effect', which intersects the horizontal axis at the point at which there is no difference between the interventions.

The result of each study is shown by a box that represents the point estimate of the outcome measure.

- The area of the box is proportional to the weight each study is given in the meta-analysis. Studies with larger samples sizes and with more precise estimates (ie tighter confidence intervals) are given more weight.

Across each box there is a horizontal line. The width of the horizontal line represents the 95% confidence interval.

- If the outcome measure on the horizontal axis is a ratio, such as the relative risk, the 95% confidence interval is asymmetrical around each study outcome. If relative risks are plotted on a logarithm scale the confidence interval will be symmetrical around each study outcome.

- If the horizontal line touches or crosses the line of no effect, either the study outcome was not statistically significant or the sample size was too small to allow us to be confident about where the true result lies (or both).

- If the horizontal line does not cross the line of no effect, the results are statistically significant.

The overall outcome of the meta-analysis is a diamond shape:

- The centre of the diamond is located at the point estimate of the pooled result.

- The horizontal width of the diamond shape is the 95% confidence interval for the overall result.

- There might be an ascending dotted line from upper corner of the diamond.

- In some forest plots the diamond shape is unfilled and the confidence interval is shown as a horizontal line through the diamond. If the confidence interval is narrow, this line might be contained within the diamond.

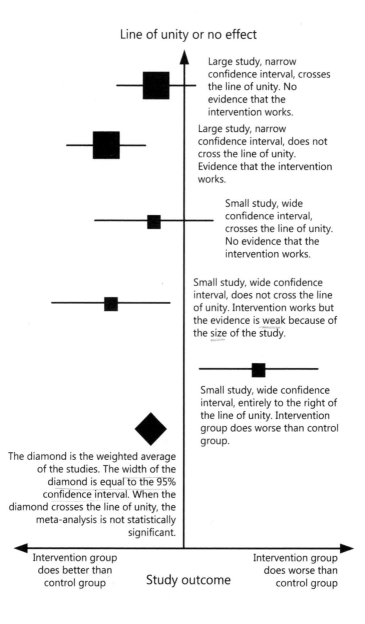

Figure 30 Understanding a forest plot

Guidelines and review libraries

The PRISMA Statement aims to help authors improve the reporting of systematic reviews and meta-analyses. PRISMA stands for Preferred Reporting Items for Systematic Reviews and Meta-Analyses. It consists of a 27-item checklist and a four-phase flow diagram. It is an evolving document that is subject to change periodically as new evidence emerges. In fact, the PRISMA Statement is an update and expansion of the now-outdated QUOROM Statement. The current definitive version of the PRISMA Statement can be found on the PRISMA website (www.prisma-statement.org/).

The **MOOSE group** (the Meta-analysis Of Observational Studies in Epidemiology) has published a checklist containing specifications for reporting of meta-analyses of observational studies in epidemiology[1]. Use of the checklist should improve the usefulness of meta-analyses for authors, reviewers, editors, readers and decision makers (www.consort-statement.org/).

PROSPERO is a prospective register of systematic reviews of health and social care interventions produced and maintained by the Centre for Reviews and Dissemination (www.crd.york.ac.uk/prospero/).

The Cochrane Collaboration, established in 1993, is an international network working to help healthcare providers, policy makers, patients and their advocates and carers make well-informed decisions about healthcare, based on the best available research evidence. The Cochrane Collaboration prepares, updates and promotes the accessibility of **Cochrane Reviews**, which are systematic reviews of primary research in human healthcare and health policy. They are published online in The Cochrane Library (www.thecochranelibrary.com/).

1   Stroup DF, Berlin JA, Morton SC, et al. Meta-analysis of observational studies in epidemiology: a proposal for reporting. Meta-analysis Of Observational Studies in Epidemiology (MOOSE) group. *JAMA* 2000, 283, 2008–12.

HETEROGENEITY AND HOMOGENEITY

Scenario 14

Randomised controlled trials comparing antidepressant treatment with placebo took place in three cities, London, Paris and Sydney. The results for London and Paris were similar. The patients in Sydney reported remarkably different results, with much bigger improvements in depressive rating scale scores. Before the results of the three centres were combined, a scrutiny of the methodology used in each centre indicated a methodological difference. In London and Paris, patients were invited to busy outpatient departments to report their progress. In Sydney, the patients were invited to a hotel suite where they were given tea and cakes while waiting for the researchers. The researchers commented that the difference in results was not due to random chance alone.

Because the aim of the meta-analysis is to summate the results of similar studies, there are tests to ensure that the studies merit combination. Any variation seen to occur between study results can be due to chance or systematic differences or both.

Homogeneity is when studies have similar and consistent results and any observed differences are due to random variation.

When there is more variation than would be expected by chance alone, even after allowing for random variation, this is referred to as **heterogeneity**.

If there is substantial heterogeneity between studies this can bias the summary effect and the summary statistic is therefore unreliable. By identifying heterogeneity you can adjust and correct the overall results before producing an overall estimate.

Heterogeneity can occur at different stages. It can occur as differences in the composition of the groups, in the design of the study or in the outcome. There might be differences, for example, in population characteristics, baseline risks, prescribing effects, clinical settings, methodological factors or outcome measures. It can also occur if the studies are small and the event rate is low, when the results for the groups can differ significantly and you cannot rely on the summary estimate.

Clinical heterogeneity occurs when the individuals chosen for two studies differ from one another significantly, making the results of these studies difficult to collate.

Statistical heterogeneity occurs when the results of the different studies differ from one another significantly more than would be expected by chance.

Summary effect size

There are two ways to calculate the effect size to summarise the results for a meta-analysis:

- **Fixed-effects model:** This assumes that there is no heterogeneity between the studies, ie that the trials are all comparable and that any differences that are present are due to the treatments themselves (homogeneity).

- **Random-effects model:** This allows for between-study variations when the pooled overall effect estimate is produced (heterogeneity).

If heterogeneity has been ruled out, a fixed-effects model is used. If heterogeneity does exist, a random-effects model is used. The random-effects model will give wider confidence intervals than fixed-effect models in the presence of significant heterogeneity.

The two types of fixed-effects models for relative risk and odds ratio used to produce a summary statistic are:

- **The Mantel–Haenszel procedure:** The most widely used statistical method for producing the final result of a forest plot. It combines the results of trials to produce a single-value overall summary of the net effect. The result is given as a chi-squared statistic associated with a *P* value.

- **The Peto method:** This is for individual and combined odds ratios. This method produces biased results in some circumstances, especially when calculated odds ratios are far from 1.

Methods to test for heterogeneity

- **Forest plot:** This provides visual evidence of heterogeneity if present. Heterogeneity is indicated if the confidence interval of a study does not overlap with any of the confidence intervals of the other studies. If the horizontal lines all overlap to some extent the trials are homogeneous.

- **Cochran's Q:** Based on the chi-squared test, Cochran's Q is calculated as the weighted sum of the squared differences of each study's estimate from the overall pooled estimate. *P* values are obtained by comparing the statistic with a chi-squared distribution with $n - 1$ degrees of freedom, where n is equal to the number of studies. Cochran's Q has low power to test heterogeneity if the number of studies is small.

- **I-squared statistic:** Indicates the proportion of the variation seen across studies that is not due to chance. It ranges in value from 0% (no heterogeneity) to 100%. Heterogeneity is considered to be present if I-squared $\geq$ 50%.

- **Z statistic:** If a Z statistic is quoted, this should be associated with a P value or confidence intervals. If $Z > 2.2$ the null hypothesis can be rejected, ie there is heterogeneity present.

- **Galbraith plot:** A Galbraith plot is useful when the number of studies is small. It is a graph with 1/SE on the X axis and the Z statistic on the Y axis. The summary effect line goes through the middle. Heterogeneity is indicated by studies lying a certain number of standard deviations above or below this summary effect line.

Some methods aim to identify homogeneity and as a result can be used to eliminate heterogeneity, eg:

- **L'Abbé plot:** This plots on the X axis the percentage with successful outcome in the control group, and on the Y axis the percentage with successful outcome in the experimental group. A diagonal line is drawn between the two axes and above the line represents effective treatment; below the line represents ineffective treatment. The more compact the distribution of the points on the graph, the more likely it is that homogeneity is present and the less likely it is that there is heterogeneity present.

In summary,

If no heterogeneity is found:

- you can perform a meta-analysis and generate a common summary effect measure, and
- decide on what data to combine
- examples of measures that can be combined include:
  o risk ratio
  o odds ratio
  o risk difference
  o effect size (Z statistic, standardised mean difference)
  o P values

o   correlation coefficient

o   sensitivity and specificity of a diagnostic test

If significant heterogeneity is found:

- you can decide not to combine the data, and
- find out what factors might explain it, using one of these approaches:

    o   graphical methods

    o   meta-regression

    o   sensitivity analysis

    o   subgroup analysis

Meta-regression analysis

Meta-regression is a method that can be used to try to adjust for heterogeneity in a meta-analysis. It can test to see whether there is evidence of different effects in different subgroups of trials. For example, you can use meta-regression to test whether treatment effects are greater in studies of low quality than in studies of high quality.

Meta-regression analysis aims to relate the size of a treatment effect to factors within a study, rather than just obtaining one summary effect across all the trials. For example, the use of statins to lower cholesterol levels may be investigated by a series of trials. A meta-analysis of these trials might produce a summary effect size across all the trials. A meta-regression analysis will provide information on the role of statin dosage and its effect on lowering cholesterol levels, helping to explain any heterogeneity of treatment effect between the studies present in the meta-analysis. Meta-regression is most useful when there is high variability in the factor being examined.

Sensitivity analysis

Sensitivity analyses assess how sensitive the results of the analysis are to changes in the way it was done. It allows researchers to see if the results would change significantly if key decisions or underlying assumptions in the set-up and methodology of the trial were changed. If the results are not significantly changed during sensitivity analyses, the researchers can be more confident of the results. If the results do change such that the conclusions drawn will also differ, researchers need to discuss these factors.

Reporting bias is the term applied to a group of related biases that can lead to over-representation of significant or positive studies in systematic reviews. Types of reporting bias include time-lag bias, language bias, citation bias, funding bias, outcome variable selection bias, developed country bias, publication bias and multiple publication bias.

Publication bias

Studies with positive findings are more likely to be submitted and published than studies with negative findings. As a result, smaller studies with negative findings tend to be omitted from meta-analyses, leading to a positive bias in the overall estimate. These positive studies are also more likely to be published in English and more likely to be cited by other authors.

If the results of these small studies differ systematically from those that are included in the systematic review, their exclusion means that the overall results are misleading. The over-representation of positive studies in systematic reviews may mean that the results are biased toward a positive result.

There are several methods available to identify publication bias, including **funnel plots**, the **Galbraith plot** (possible publication bias is indicated by a positive intercept for the regression line, which should pass through the origin), and tests such as the **Egger's test**, **Begg's rank correlation test** and **Rosenthal's fail-safe N**.

Funnel plots

Funnel plots are scatter plots of treatment effects estimated from individual studies (on the X axis) and some measure of study size on the Y axis. The shape of the funnel depends on what is plotted on the Y axis (**Figure 31**).

The variables on the Y axis can include any of the following:

- Standard error
- Precision (1/standard error)
- Sample size
- 1/sample size
- log(sample size)
- log(1/sample size)

The statistical power of a trial is determined by both the sample size and the number of patients who develop the event. This is why the standard error as the measure of study size is a good choice. Also, plotting against precision (1/ standard error) emphasises differences between larger studies.

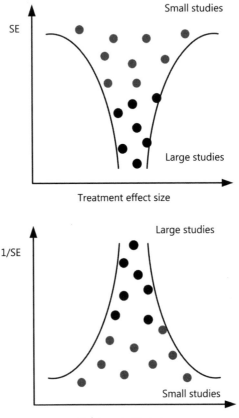

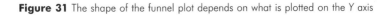

Figure 31 The shape of the funnel plot depends on what is plotted on the Y axis

Each point on the graph represents one of the studies. Precision in estimating the underlying treatment effect increases as a study's sample size increases. This means that effect estimates from small studies scatter more widely at the open end (the widest part) of the funnel. Larger studies have greater precision and provide more similar measures of effect that are nearer to the true effect, and these will lie at the narrow end of the funnel.

Asymmetry of funnel plots

In the absence of bias, the plot therefore resembles a symmetrical funnel. If there is publication bias, there will be asymmetry of the open/wide end due to the absence of small negative results (**Figure 32**). Asymmetry might also be due to the tendency for the smaller studies to show larger treatment effects and heterogeneity between trials. The overall estimate of treatment effect from a meta-analysis should be examined closely if there is asymmetry of a funnel plot.

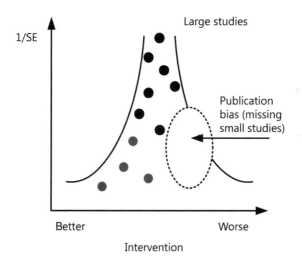

Figure 32 A funnel plot can reveal publication bias

The **'trim and fill' method** can be used with funnel plots to correct for publication bias. First, the number of 'asymmetrical' trials on one side of the funnel is estimated. These trials are then removed, or 'trimmed' from the funnel, leaving a symmetrical remainder from which the true centre of the funnel is estimated by standard meta-analysis procedures. The trimmed trials are then replaced and their missing counterparts 'filled': these are mirror images of the trimmed trials with the mirror axis placed at the pooled estimate. This then allows an adjusted overall confidence interval to be calculated. Other methods used to detect funnel-plot asymmetry include the regression method and the rank correlation approach.

INTERIM ANALYSIS

Trials can take several months from start to finish. Interim analyses allow researchers to see the results at specific time points before the end of the study. Interim analyses can help to identify flaws in the study design and can help in identifying significant beneficial or harmful effects that may be occurring. This can sometimes result in the study being stopped early for ethical reasons if it is clear that one group is receiving treatment that is more harmful or less beneficial than another.

There is a potential problem with interim analyses. If multiple analyses are performed, positive findings might arise solely by chance and mislead the researchers into making a type 1 error. Several statistical methods are available to adjust for multiple analyses. Their use should be specified in the trial protocol.

In March 2009 Pfizer stopped a randomised placebo-controlled trial of its drug Sutent (sunitinib) in patients with pancreatic islet cell tumours. The trial began in 2007 and was expected to be completed in 2011. The primary measure of effectiveness was progression-free survival, or time until death or disease progression. An independent data-monitoring committee recommended stopping the trial early after it concluded the drug improved progression-free survival versus placebo. All patients were given the option to continue taking Sutent or be switched from placebo to Sutent.

In April 2009 Pfizer stopped a phase 3 trial comparing its drug Sutent (sunitinib) with Xeloda (capecitabine) in the treatment of advanced breast cancer. The primary endpoint was progression-free survival. An independent monitoring committee found that Sutent was unlikely to prove better as a stand-alone treatment than Xeloda among patients who had not previously benefited from standard treatments.

SECTION D

USING CHECKLISTS

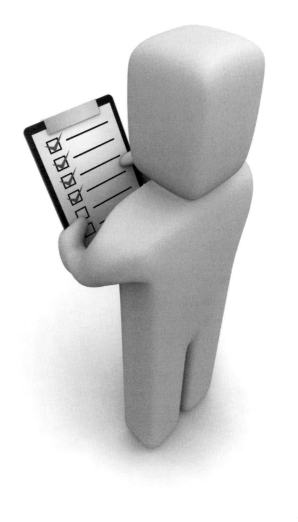

INTRODUCTION TO CHECKLISTS

All clinical papers can be understood and critically appraised using the structure that we have described so far. The clinical question and study type are considered before the methodology and results are appraised.

Research work can be classified by the type of study design used and also by the subject area of the clinical question. For example, some studies look at aetiological factors; others look at the usefulness of diagnostic tests. Within different clinical areas, there might be specific questions to ask, particularly with regard to the methodology and results. Applicability concerns tend to be the same.

Checklists provide a way to work through the key considerations when critically appraising different study types, by listing the key points in the methodology, reporting of results and applicability. Many institutions have published checklists, but the most highly acclaimed checklists were published in the *Users' Guides to the Medical Literature* series, published between 1993 and 2000 in the *Journal of the American Medical Association* (*JAMA*) by the Evidence-Based Medicine Working Group (see the 'Further reading' chapter on page 218).

The chapters in this section give a concise overview of the checklists that we use in our clinical practice. To avoid duplication, we will only elaborate on new terms and concepts.

AETIOLOGICAL STUDIES

Aetiological studies compare the risk of developing an outcome in one or more groups exposed to one or more risk factors (**Figure 33, Table 28**). Study types commonly used include case–control and cohort studies.

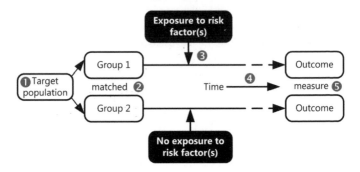

Figure 33 Aetiological studies (the numbered steps in the methodology are explained in **Table 28**)

METHODOLOGY

here a clearly defined group of patients? (1)
pt for the exposure studied, were the groups similar to each other? (2)
the exposure precede the onset of the outcome? (3)
s the follow-up of the subjects complete and of sufficient duration? (4)
re exposures and clinical outcomes measured in the same way in both groups? (5)

RESULTS

elative risk in a randomised trial or cohort study
Odds ratio in a case–control study
Precision of the estimate of risk – confidence limits
Is there a dose–response gradient? → why is this important?
Does the association make biological sense?

APPLICABILITY

Are your patients similar to the target population?
Are the risk factor(s) similar to those experienced in your population?
What are your patients' risks of the adverse outcome (number needed to harm)?
Should exposure to the risk factor(s) be stopped or minimised?

Table 28 Aetiological studies checklist (the numbers relate to the study pathway outlined in **Figure 33**)

A diagnostic study compares a new test for diagnosing a condition with the gold-standard method (**Figure 34, Table 29**).

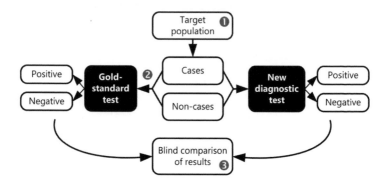

Figure 34 Diagnostic studies (the numbered steps in the methodology are explained in **Table 29**)

A good test will correctly identify patients with the condition (**true positives**) while minimising the number of patients without the condition who also test positive (**false positives**). Similarly, it will correctly identify patients who do not have the condition (**true negatives**) and minimise the number of patients given negative results when they do have the condition (**false negatives**).

Screening tests look for the early signs of a disease in asymptomatic people so that the disease can be treated before it gets to an advanced stage. The acceptability of false-positive and false-negative results depends in part on the seriousness of the condition and its treatment. A false-positive result causes unnecessary anxiety for the patient and can lead to expensive, unpleasant or dangerous treatments that are not indicated. A false-negative result on the other hand can lull a patient into a false sense of security and other symptoms and signs of disease might be ignored.

METHODOLOGY

Did the patient sample include an appropriate spectrum of patients to whom the test will be applied? (1)
Was the gold standard applied regardless of the diagnostic test result? (2)
Was there was an independent and blind comparison with a gold standard of diagnosis? (3)

RESULTS

Sensitivity
Specificity
Positive predictive value
Negative predictive value
Likelihood ratios
Pre-test probability and odds
Post-test probability and odds
Receiver operating curve

APPLICABILITY

Are your patients similar to the target population?
Is it possible to integrate this test into your clinical settings and procedures?
Who will carry out the test in your clinical setting and who will interpret the results?
Will the results of the test affect your management of the patient?
Is the test affordable?

Table 29 Diagnostic or screening studies checklist (the numbers relate to the study pathway outlined in **Figure 34**)

Characteristics of the test

The results of the comparison of a diagnostic test with a gold-standard test need to be tabulated in a 2 × 2 table, as shown in **Table 30**. Note that each subject needs to take **two** diagnostic tests – the gold-standard test and the new test. The values of a, b, c and d will either be given or can be deduced from other data given in the results section.

		DISEASE STATUS BY GOLD STANDARD		
		positive	negative	Totals
DISEASE STATUS BY DIAGNOSTIC TEST	positive	a	b	a + b
	negative	c	d	c + d
Totals		a + c	b + d	a + b + c + d

Table 30 A 2 × 2 table for the results of diagnostic tests

There are a number of words and phrases used to describe the characteristics of a diagnostic test (**Table 31**). Each of these values should be calculated. A learning aid to help remember the formulae is shown in **Figure 35**.

TEST CHARACTERISTICS	DESCRIPTION	FORMULA
Sensitivity (true-positive rate)	The proportion of subjects with the disorder (by gold standard) who have a positive result (by new test)	$\dfrac{a}{a + c}$
Specificity (true-negative rate)	The proportion of subjects who do not have the disorder and who have a negative test	$\dfrac{d}{b + d}$
Positive predictive value (PPV)	The proportion of subjects who have a positive test result who do have the disorder	$\dfrac{a}{a + b}$

Negative predictive value (NPV)	The proportion of subjects with a negative test result who do not have the illness	$\dfrac{d}{c + d}$
Likelihood ratio for a positive test result (LR+)	How much more likely is a positive test to be found in a person with, as opposed to without, the condition?	$\dfrac{\text{sensitivity}}{1 - \text{specificity}}$
Likelihood ratio for a negative test result (LR–)	How much more likely is a negative test to be found in a person with, as opposed to without, the condition?	$\dfrac{1 - \text{sensitivity}}{\text{specificity}}$
Accuracy of a test	The proportion of subjects given the correct result	$(a + d) / (a + b + c + d)$

Table 31 Diagnostic test characteristics

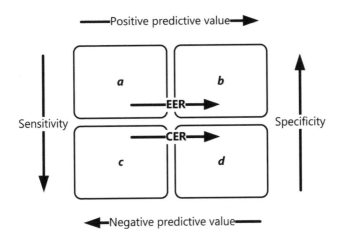

Figure 35 Learning aid for the characteristics of a diagnostic test. For example, the arrow for sensitivity starts at box *a* and goes over boxes *a* and *c*; sensitivity therefore equals *a* / (*a* + *c*). EER = experimental event rate; CER = control event rate (see page 94).

There are also a number of risks and odds that can be calculated for the patient (**Table 32**).

PATIENT RISKS & ODDS	DESCRIPTION	FORMULA
Pre-test probability (equivalent to prevalence)	The probability that a subject will have the disorder	$$\frac{a + c}{a + b + c + d}$$
Pre-test odds	The odds that a subject will have the disorder	$$\frac{\text{pre-test probability}}{1 - \text{pre-test probability}}$$
Post-test odds	The odds that a subject, scoring positive on the diagnostic test, actually has the disorder	pre-test odds x $LR+$
Post-test probability	The probability that a subject, scoring positive on the diagnostic test, actually has the disorder	$$\frac{\text{post-test odds}}{\text{post-test odds} + 1}$$

Table 32 Patient risks and odds

Understanding results

Sensitivity, specificity and predictive values can be confusing. The following statements clarify the difference between sensitivity and positive predictive value:

- **Sensitivity:** If a patient has a disorder, what is the chance of getting a positive result on the new test?
- **Positive predictive value:** If a patient has a positive result on the new test, what is the chance that they do have the disorder?

The following statements clarify the difference between specificity and negative predictive value:

- **Specificity:** If a patient does not have the disorder, what is the chance of getting a negative result on the new test?
- **Negative predictive value:** If a patient has a negative result on the new test, what is the chance that they do not have the disorder?

The sensitivity and specificity of a test can be interpreted using the following statements and aides-mémoires:

- **SpPin** – when a highly **sp**ecific test is used, a **p**ositive test result tends to rule **in** the disorder.
- **SnNout** – when a highly **sen**sitive test is used, a **n**egative test result tends to rule **out** the disorder.

The sensitivity and specificity are not affected by changes in the prevalence of the disorder.

Predictive values depend on the prevalence of the disorder and will change as the disorder becomes rarer in the population:

- Positive predictive value will decrease.
- Negative predictive value will increase.
- Post-test probabilities also change.

Likelihood ratios are more useful than predictive values. As likelihood ratios are calculated from sensitivity and specificity, they remain constant even when the prevalence of the disorder changes, unlike predictive values.

Likelihood ratios show how many times more likely patients with a disorder are to have a particular test result than patients without the disorder.

- The likelihood ratio for a positive test result should be as high as possible above 1. Positive results are desirable in patients with the disorder.

- The likelihood ratio for a negative test result should be as low as possible below 1. Negative test results are undesirable in patients with the disorder.

The likelihood ratio nomogram (or 'Fagan nomogram') enables the post-test probability to be graphically calculated if the pre-test probability and likelihood ratio are known (**Figure 36**). If a line is drawn connecting the pre-test probability of disease and the likelihood ratio, it intersects at the post-test probability of disease when extended to the right.

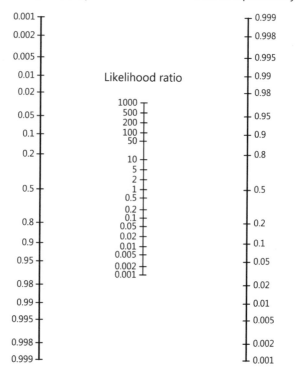

Figure 36 Likelihood ratio nomogram

The performance of a diagnostic test often varies from one clinical location to another and the interpretation of results might also differ. This needs to be considered when deciding the applicability of any research findings.

Multiple testing

Serial testing (eg diagnosing HIV – if a first test is positive, another test is done to confirm) increases specificity (the true-negative rate).

Parallel testing (eg diagnosing myocardial infarction – history, ECG, enzymes) increases sensitivity (the true-positive rate).

Receiver operating characteristic (ROC) curve

There is a threshold with any diagnostic test above which a positive result is returned and below which a negative result is returned. During the development of a diagnostic test, this threshold can be varied to assess the trade-off between sensitivity and specificity. With any change in the cut-off point the sensitivity can increase and the specificity can decrease, or vice versa.

A good diagnostic test would, ideally, be one that has low false-positive and false-negative rates. A bad diagnostic test is one in which the only cut-offs that make the false-positive rate low lead to a high false-negative rate and vice versa. To find the optimum cut-off point, a **receiver operating characteristic curve** is used. This is a graphical representation of the relationship between the false-negative and false-positive rates for each cut-off. The plot shows the false-positive rate (1 – specificity) on the X axis and the true-positive rate (sensitivity or 1 – false-negative rate) on the Y axis (**Figure 37**).

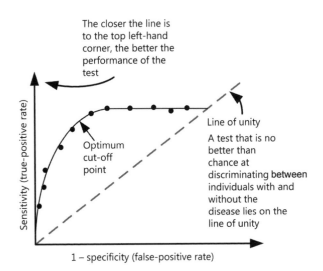

Figure 37 Receiver operating curve

The **area under the curve** represents the probability that the test will correctly identify true-positive and true-negative results. An area of 1 represents a perfect test, whereas an area of 0.5 represents a worthless test.

The more closely the curve follows the left-hand border and then the top border of the receiver operating curve space, the more accurate the test – the true-positive rate is high and the false-positive rate is low. This is the point where the area under the curve is the greatest. The best cut-off point is the point at which the curve is closest to the top left-hand corner.

If two different tests or continuous variables are plotted on the same receiver operating characteristic curve, the test or variable with the curve that lies above the curve of the other test or variable is the better choice. It will have the greatest area under the curve.

STARD statement

The objective of the STARD initiative (STAndards for the Reporting of Diagnostic accuracy studies) is to improve the accuracy and completeness of reporting of studies of diagnostic accuracy. The STARD statement consists of a checklist of 25 items that can viewed on their website (www.stard-statement.org/).

Self-assessment exercise 14

1. A new test is developed to test for diabetes mellitus. A gold-standard blood test diagnoses 33 people as diabetic out of a study population of 136. The new test diagnoses 34 people as positive, including two people who were not diagnosed by the gold-standard test.

    a. What are the sensitivity, specificity, positive predictive value and negative predictive value for the test?

    b. What are the likelihood ratios for positive and negative test results?

    c. What are the pre-test and post-test probabilities and odds?

TREATMENT STUDIES

Treatment studies compare the effects of a new intervention with those of another intervention (**Figure 38, Table 33**). A good intervention will improve the outcome compared with previously available interventions. The improvement can be stated in absolute terms, in relative terms or by the number needed to treat (NNT).

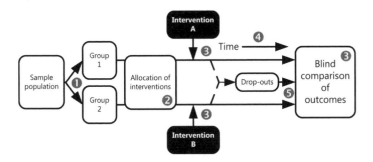

Figure 38 Treatment studies (the numbered steps in the methodology are explained in **Table 33**)

METHODOLOGY
Was there a clearly focused clinical question and primary hypothesis?
Was the randomisation process clearly explained? (1)
Were the groups similar at the start of the study?
Was concealed allocation used in the allocation of interventions? (2)
Were the groups treated equally apart from the experimental intervention?
Was blinding used effectively? (3)
Was follow-up complete and of sufficient duration? (4)
Was this an intention-to-treat study? (5)

RESULTS
Control event rate
Experimental event rate
Absolute risk reduction / benefit increase
Relative risk reduction / benefit increase
Numbers needed to treat
Precision of the estimate of treatment effect – confidence limits

APPLICABILITY
Are your patients similar to the target population? Were all the relevant outcome factors considered? Will the intervention help your patients? Are the benefits of the intervention worth the risks and costs? Have patients' values and preferences been considered?

Table 33 Treatment studies checklist (the numbers relate to the study pathway outlined in **Figure 38**)

Translating NNT to your own patient population

The numbers needed to treat (NNT) calculated in a study might not directly reflect what will happen in a clinical population, where there are many more factors to consider. There are three principal methods available for estimating the NNT for patients in a clinical setting:

- **F:** This requires that you estimate your patient's risk compared with that the control group from the study. If your patient is twice as susceptible as those in the trial, $F = 2$ for example. The NNT for your patient is simply the trial's reported NNT divided by F, assuming the treatment produces the same relative risk reduction for patients at different levels of risk:

$$\text{NNT for your patient} = \text{NNT}/F$$

- **PEER:** Alternatively, you could start from an estimate of your patient's risk of an event (patient expected event rate or PEER) without the treatment. This estimate could be based on the study's control group or on other prognostic evidence, but you should use your clinical judgement. Multiply this PEER by the relative risk reduction (RRR) for the study: the result is your patient's absolute risk reduction (ARR), from which the NNT for your patient can be calculated:

$$\text{NNT} = 1 / (\text{PEER} \times \text{RRR})$$

or

$$\text{NNH} = 1 / (\text{PEER} \times \text{RRI})$$

  o We assume that the same relative benefit would apply to patients at different levels of risk.

  o **Bayes' theorem:** Use a treatment nomogram for Bayes' theorem.

PROGNOSTIC STUDIES

A prognostic study examines the characteristics of the patient that might predict any of the possible outcomes (prognostic factors) and the likelihood that different outcome events will occur (**Figure 39**, **Table 34**). Outcomes can be positive or negative events. The likelihood of different outcomes occurring can be expressed absolutely, relatively or in the form of a survival curve.

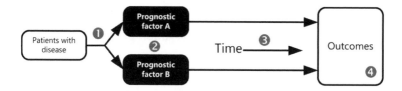

Figure 39 Prognostic studies (the numbered steps in the methodology are explained in **Table 34**)

METHODOLOGY
Was a sample of patients recruited at a common point in the course of the disease? (1) Was there adjustment for important prognostic factors? (2) Was follow-up complete and of sufficient duration? (3) Was there blind assessment of objective outcome criteria? (4)
RESULTS
Absolute risk – eg 5-year survival rate Relative risk – eg risk from a prognostic factor Survival curves – cumulative events over time Precision of the prognostic estimates – confidence limits
APPLICABILITY
Are your patients similar to the patients in this study? Does this study give you a better understanding of the progress of disease and the possible outcomes? Does this study help you to decide whether to reassure or counsel your patients?

Table 34 Prognostic studies checklist (the numbers relate to the study pathway outlined in **Figure 39**)

Survival analysis

Survival analysis studies the time between entry into a study and a subsequent occurrence of an event. Originally, such analyses were performed to give information on time to death in fatal conditions, but they can be applied to many other outcomes as well as mortality.

Survival analysis is usually applied to data from longitudinal cohort studies. There are, however, problems when analysing data relating to the time between one event and another:

- All times to the event occurring will differ, but it is unlikely that these times will be normally distributed.
- The subjects might not all have entered the study at the same time, so there are **unequal observation periods**.
- Some patients might not reach the endpoint by the end of the study. For example, if the event is recovery within 12 months, some patients might not have recovered in the 12-month study period.
- Patients can leave a study early, not experience the event or be lost to follow-up. The data for these individuals are referred to as **censored**.

Both censored observations and unequal observation periods make it difficult to determine the mean survival times because we do not have all the survival times. As a result, the curve is used to calculate the **median survival time**.

Median survival time

Median survival time is the time from the start of the study that coincides with a 50% probability of survival – that is, the time taken for 50% of the subjects not to have had the event. This value is associated with a P value and 95% confidence intervals.

Kaplan–Meier survival analysis

The Kaplan–Meier survival analysis looks at event rates over the study period, rather than just at a specific time point. It is used to determine survival probabilities and proportions of individuals surviving, enabling the estimation of a cumulative survival probability. The data are presented in life tables and survival curves (**Figure 40**).

The data are first ranked in ascending order over time in life tables. The survival curve is plotted by calculating the proportion of patients who remain alive in the study each time an event occurs, taking into account censored observations. The survival curve will not change at the time of censoring, but only when the next event occurs. Censored patients are assumed to have the same survival prospects as those who continue in the study.

Time is plotted on the X axis, and the proportion of people without the outcome (survivors) at each time point are plotted on the Y axis. A cumulative curve is achieved, with steps at each time an event occurs. Small vertical ticks on the curve indicate the times at which patients are censored.

A survival curve can be used to calculate several parameters:

* The **median survival time**, which is the time taken until 50% of the population survive
* The **survival time**, which is the time taken for a certain proportion of the population to survive
* The **survival probability** at a given time point, which is the probability that an individual will not have developed an endpoint event

A survival curve can also be used to compare the difference in the proportions surviving in two groups and their confidence intervals, such as when comparing a control population with an experimental population.

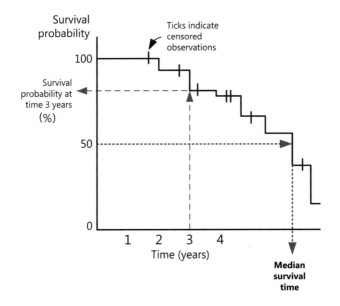

Figure 40 Survival curve

Log-rank test

To compare the survival experiences of two or more populations, the proportions of people surviving in each population at any given time point can be compared. This snapshot does not, however, reflect the total survival experience of the two groups.

The **log-rank test** is a better method as it takes the entire follow-up period into account. It is a significance test and helps to decide whether or not to accept the null hypothesis that there is no difference in the probability of survival in the different groups. It does not indicate the size of the difference between the groups, unlike the hazard ratio.

The log-rank test is so called because the data are first ranked and then compared with observations and expected outcome rates in each of the groups (similar to a chi-squared test). The log-rank test does not take other variables into consideration.

Hazard

The **hazard rate** is the probability of an endpoint event in a time interval divided by the duration of the time interval. The hazard rate can be interpreted as the instantaneous probability of an endpoint event in a study if the time interval is short. The hazard rate might not be constant during the study.

The **hazard ratio** is the hazard rate in the experimental arm divided by the hazard rate of the control arm. The hazard ratio is complemented by a P value and confidence intervals. It is assumed that the hazard ratio remains constant throughout the study.

- If the hazard ratio is 1, the two arms have an equal hazard rate.
- If the hazard ratio is > 1, the experimental arm has an increased hazard.
- If the hazard ratio is < 1, the experimental arm has a reduced hazard.

Although the interpretation of hazard ratio is similar to that of relative risk and the odds ratio, the terms are not synonymous. The hazard ratio compares the experimental and control groups throughout the study duration, unlike the relative risk and odds ratio, which only compare the proportion of subjects that achieved the outcome in each group at the end of the study.

It is not possible to calculate the hazard ratio from a 2×2 contingency table.

Cox proportional hazards regression is used to produce the hazard ratio. It is the multivariate extension of the log-rank test. It is used to assess the impact of treatment on survival or other time-related events and adjusts for the effects of other variables.

Resources within the NHS are finite. Not every activity can be funded. Economic analyses evaluate the choices in resource allocation by comparing the costs and consequences of different actions. They tend to take a wider perspective on healthcare provision than other types of studies, because they do not just focus on whether one intervention is statistically better than another. They aim to discover which interventions can be used to produce the maximum possible benefits.

Economic analyses can be appraised in much the same way as other types of studies (**Table 35**). All direct, indirect and intangible costs and benefits should be included in a good economic analysis. Much of the debate regarding economic analyses tends to focus on the assumptions made in order to calculate monetary values for the use of resources and the consequent benefits. Such assumptions are based on large amounts of information collected from different sources, including demographic data, epidemiological data, socioeconomic data and the economic burden of disease.

METHODOLOGY
Is there a full economic comparison of healthcare strategies?
Does it identify all other costs and effects?
Were the costs and outcomes properly measured and valued?
Were appropriate allowances made for uncertainties in the analysis?
Are the costs and outcomes related to the baseline risk in the treatment population?

RESULTS
Incremental costs and outcomes of each strategy
Cost-minimisation analysis
Cost-effectiveness analysis
Cost–utility analysis
Cost–benefit analysis

APPLICABILITY
Can I use this study in caring for my patients?
Could my patients expect similar outcomes?
Do the costs apply in my own setting?
Are the conclusions unlikely to change with modest changes in costs and outcomes?

Table 35 Economic studies checklist

A subdiscipline of health economics is pharmacoeconomics. This refers to the scientific method that compares the value of one drug with the value of another. A pharmacoeconomic study evaluates the cost (expressed in monetary terms) and effects (expressed in terms of monetary value, efficacy or enhanced quality of life) of a drug.

Examples of input costs:

- Direct medical costs – hospitalisations, equipment and facilities, medical and nursing time, drugs and dressings
- Direct non-medical costs – out-of-pocket expenses, time costs, volunteer time
- Indirect costs – productivity changes
- Intangible costs – quality of life, pain, suffering

Examples of output benefits:

- Associated economic effects – direct medical savings, direct non-medical savings, indirect savings, intangible savings
- Natural units (health effects) – endpoints, surrogate endpoints, survival
- Utility units (preference-weighted effects) – health status, quality of life

There are several types of economic evaluation and they differ in which consequences they measure.

Cost-of-illness study

This is not a true economic evaluation in fact, because it does not compare the costs and outcomes of alternative courses of action. It actually measures all the costs that are associated with a particular condition and these can include some of the following:

- Direct costs – where real money is actually changing hands, eg health service use
- Indirect costs – costs that are not directly accountable to a particular function, eg the costs of lost productivity from time taken off work due to the condition
- Intangible costs – the costs associated with the disvalue to a patient of pain and suffering

Cost-minimisation analysis

This analysis is used when interventions are being compared which produce the same beneficial outcome and the benefit is of the same order of magnitude (**Figure 41**).

- Example: The treatment of headache using paracetamol or aspirin

The analysis simply aims to decide the least costly way of achieving the same outcome. Any difference in outcome is not taken into consideration.

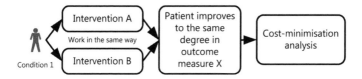

Figure 41 Cost-minimisation analysis

Cost-effectiveness analysis (CEA)

This type of analysis is used in situations where the outcome is the same for the alternative interventions but achieved by different mechanisms and to different degrees (**Figure 42**). The amount of improvement therefore has to be factored in to the economic analysis as well as the cost of the interventions. Only one outcome is considered.

- Example: The treatment of back pain using physiotherapy or surgery

The cost-effectiveness of an intervention is the ratio of the cost of the intervention to the improvement in the outcome measure, which is expressed in non-monetary units (eg the number of pain-free days). The cost-effectiveness of an intervention is only meaningful when compared with other interventions.

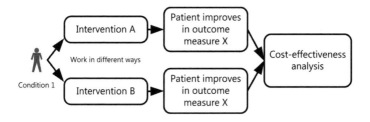

Figure 42 Cost-effectiveness analysis

Cost–consequences analysis

Cost–consequences analysis is a form of cost-effectiveness analysis for situations where there is more than one outcome measure. Instead of combining several outcomes to create a single index of health utility, in a cost–consequence analysis all outcomes are presented with relevant cost-effectiveness ratios, and the reader can judge the relative importance of the outcomes.

Cost–utility analysis

A cost–utility analysis is used to make choices between interventions for different conditions in which the units of outcome differ (**Figure 43**). Cost–utility analysis is better than cost-effectiveness analysis in situations where interventions give outcomes that are not perfect health.

- Example: The treatment of breast cancer using a new drug versus hip replacement surgery

As the outcomes cannot be directly compared, a common unit or **utility measure** (which is indicative of both the quantity and quality of life afterwards) is used.

The best known utility measure is the **quality-adjusted life year** or QALY.

$$QALY = (\text{number of extra years of} \times (\text{the value of the quality of} \\ \text{life obtained}) \qquad \text{life during those extra years})$$

In terms of the quality of life over 1 year, death is equal to 0 QALYs and 1 year of perfect health is 1 QALY. The competing interventions are compared in terms of cost per utility (cost per QALY).

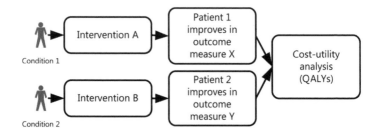

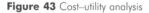

Figure 43 Cost–utility analysis

Example of a cost–utility analysis

A patient needs life-saving treatment.

- Intervention A costs £1000 and gives a patient 10 additional years of life with a quality of life of 0.2. This is equal to $10 \times 0.2 = 2$ QALYs. The cost of each QALY is £500.

- Intervention B costs £2160 and gives a patient three additional years of life with a quality of life of 0.9. This is equal to $3 \times 0.9 = 2.7$ QALYs. The cost of each QALY is £800.

- Over 10 years, Intervention B gives 0.7 additional QALYs over Intervention A.

There are two ways in which this result can influence practice:

1. If the clinician wants to offer the intervention that offers the highest number of QALYs, Intervention B is the treatment of choice. The patient might disagree and want to live longer, even if their life is harder.

2. If the clinician wants to offer the intervention that offers best value for money for the health service, Intervention A is the treatment of choice. The patient might disagree and want a better quality of life, even if their life is shorter.

Cost–benefit analysis

This analysis is used to compare the costs and benefits of different treatments for different patient groups by putting a **monetary value** on the outcomes resulting from each alternative intervention (**Figure 44**). The results for each intervention are expressed as the ratio of economic benefits to costs or as net economic benefit (ie benefits minus costs). A cost–benefit analysis for a single intervention can be considered on its own so a comparison intervention is not always necessary.

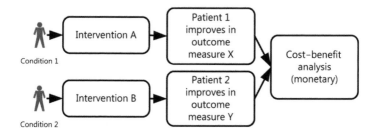

Figure 44 Cost–benefit analysis

Cost–benefit analysis considers the **opportunity cost** of a treatment choice rather than just the direct cost. Using a resource prevents it from being used in some other way. For example, if an intervention is chosen, as well as the direct cost of the intervention itself one has to consider the foregone benefits that may have been gained from choosing an alternative intervention. Only if the costs and benefits associated with the chosen intervention outweigh those of the alternative intervention should the decision to spend go ahead.

Sensitivity analysis

Economic evaluations are models based on assumptions and estimates, and aim to capture and summarise what happens in reality. Sensitivity analysis assists in assessing how robust the conclusions are, considering that there will be a degree of uncertainty about some elements of any economic analysis. It tests the consistency of the results by repeating the comparison between inputs and consequences, while varying the assumptions used. The figures are adjusted to account for the full range of possible influences.

A **one-way sensitivity analysis** changes the value of one parameter at a time.

A **multi-way sensitivity analysis** alters two or more parameters simultaneously to show the effect of combined changes.

A **probabilistic sensitivity analysis** looks at the effect on the results of an evaluation when the underlying parameters are allowed to vary simultaneously across a range according to predefined distributions. The results that this kind of analysis produces represent a more realistic estimate of uncertainty. Techniques such as a Monte Carlo simulation have been developed.

In contrast to the objective counting and measuring approach of quantitative research, qualitative research concerns itself with the subjective measurement of the processes that underlie behavioural patterns. It can investigate meanings, attitudes, beliefs, preferences and behaviours. It aims to provide complex textual descriptions instead of statistical analyses. Unlike the artificial experiments of quantitative research, the focus of qualitative research is on natural settings. Context is important, making the results less generalisable.

Qualitative research relies on inductive reasoning processes. Few assumptions are made in advance of the study. Data are used to generate theories. This is the opposite of the deductive inquiry processes seen in quantitative research, where data are used to confirm or refute a hypothesis.

Qualitative research helps doctors to understand people and the social and cultural contexts within which they live, and there has been an increasing recognition over recent years of the important role such research can play in the formation and development of medical services. Qualitative methods help to bridge the gap between scientific evidence and clinical practice and help doctors to understand the barriers to using evidence-based medicine and its limitations in informing decisions about treatment.

A checklist approach can be applied to the evaluation of qualitative research (**Table 36**). As with other types of research, a qualitative study should start with a clearly formulated question that addresses a specific clinical problem and that is amenable to investigation by qualitative methods. Examination of the research question takes place in a natural setting where the patient might normally be.

METHODOLOGY
Did the paper describe an important clinical problem?
Was a qualitative approach appropriate?
Was the setting clearly described?
How were the participants chosen?
Was the data collection comprehensive and detailed?
Were the data collected in a way that addresses the research issue?
Is there a relationship between researchers and participants that needs consideration?

RESULTS
Was the data analysis sufficiently rigorous?
Were the data analysed appropriately?
Were any quantitative methods used appropriately?
Are the results credible and repeatable?
Is there a clear statement of the findings?

APPLICABILITY
Are your patients similar to the patients in this study?
Do the results help you to understand your medical practice and outcomes better?
Does the study help you to understand your relationship with your patients and carers better?

Table 36 Qualitative research checklist

Approaches

Grounded theory: Qualitative researchers do not usually start with a theory which they aim to test. Instead, a theory is developed from the data as they are collected. The theory is said to be 'grounded' in the data. The theory is updated as new data are collected and compared with existing data. The outcome is a theory which explains the phenomenon that is under investigation.

Phenomenological: Aims to answer the question, 'What is the meaning of one's lived experience?' The researcher seeks subjects who are willing to describe their thoughts, feelings and interpretations that are related to the phenomenon under investigation.

Ethnographic: Aims to learn from (rather than to study) members of a community in order to describe and interpret a cultural or social group or system.

Historical: Aims to explain present events and anticipate future events by collecting and evaluating data about past events.

Sampling methods

Purposive: The selection of subjects who have knowledge or experience of the area being investigated. One of the most common sampling strategies.

Quota: A type of purposive sampling. Quotas are set for subjects with certain characteristics. This allows the researchers to focus on those people most likely to be able to help.

Convenience: The selection of subjects based on accessibility, ease, speed and/or low cost. Anyone who might be able to offer an insight into the phenomenon under study is selected if they are available.

Snowball: Researchers identify subjects, who are then used to refer researchers on to other subjects in their social network. This provides a means of gaining access to people who would not be readily available to take part in a study, such as those living on the periphery of society. This is also known as 'chain-referral sampling'.

Sample size

Data saturation: Researchers continue to collect data until they are no longer hearing or seeing new information.

Data gathering

Participant observation: The researcher not only observes a group but adopts a role within the group from which to participate in some manner, usually over an extended period of time. This method allows for data to be collected on naturally occurring behaviours in their usual contexts. There can be a conflict between a researcher's dual role as a researcher and a participant. An added danger is that the researcher might end up over-identifying with the group, impairing analytical objectivity.

Focus groups: The researcher interviews groups of people with something in common. The people are free to talk to each other in the group. The data arise out of the interaction between group members, rather than from interaction between the researcher and the group. Focus groups can provide data on the cultural norms of the group and are helpful for exploratory research into issues of concern to the group. However, focus groups are not naturalistic, the discussions can be dominated by some participants and there are issues around confidentiality.

In-depth interviews:

- **Structured interviews** aim to focus on certain areas in order to find answers to predetermined questions. The interviewer is in control so this technique is less naturalistic.
- **Semi-structured interviews** follow a topic guide but allow for open-ended answers and follow-up of points raised.
- **Unstructured interviews** aim to discuss a limited number of topics in great depth, with no structure or preconceived plan. The interviewee is in control.

Documents: The researcher or subject keeps a personal diary account of events, interactions, discussions and/or emotions. Official documents and questionnaires might be used.

Role-play: Subjects can be asked to give their personal feedback after playing a role or observing role-play.

Minimising bias
Complete objectivity is neither achievable nor necessarily desirable in qualitative research.

Reflexivity: The researcher acknowledges the central role they play in the research process. There is an understanding of the bidirectional effect the researcher might have had on the research findings.

Bracketing: The identification and temporary setting aside of the researcher's assumptions.

Validating data
A number of techniques are available to researchers to minimise the biases and problems that arise with qualitative studies.

Member checks: The subject confirms whether the researcher has accurately recorded data. This can be done during the interview process itself or at the end of the study. This is also known as 'informant feedback' or 'respondent validation'.

Triangulation: Data are cross-verified using more than two different sources.

Analysing data

Constant comparison analysis: This strategy involves taking individual data as they are collected and comparing them to all the other data collected, in order to make tentative conclusions, hypotheses and themes. Initial ideas and concepts are tested and new data sources are found in order to develop a grounded theory.

Content analysis: Documents, text or speech are examined to see what themes emerge. Many words of text are compressed into fewer content categories based on explicit coding rules.

GUIDELINES

Clinical guidelines aim to improve clinical effectiveness and efficiency. They assist clinicians and patients by using a combination of research evidence, clinical experience and expert opinion to recommend assessment and management strategies for patients in specific clinical situations. As most recommendations are based on high-quality research such as systematic reviews and meta-analyses, guidelines can help clinicians keep up to date with the medical literature and improve communication with patients.

Many local, national and international organisations produce clinical guidelines. However, guidelines vary in quality. They need to be critically appraised just like individual research studies. There can be issues with the process of guideline development as well as the choice and interpretation of evidence used to support recommendations.

Guideline development

1. Confirm a need for the proposed clinical guideline.
2. Identify individuals and stakeholders who will help develop the guideline.
3. Identify the evidence for the guideline.
4. Evaluate current practice against the evidence.
5. Write the guideline.
6. Agree how change will be introduced into practice.
7. Engage in consultation and peer review and amend guideline if necessary.
8. Gain ratification.
9. Implement and disseminate the guideline.
10. Audit the effectiveness of the guideline.

Appraising guidelines

AGREE

The Appraisal of Guidelines Research & Evaluation (AGREE) Instrument provides a framework for assessing the quality of clinical practice guidelines (available at www.agreecollaboration.org). The AGREE Instrument assesses both the quality of the reporting and the quality of some aspects of the recommendations. It provides an assessment of the predicted validity of a guideline, ie the likelihood that it will achieve its intended outcome. It does not assess the impact of a guideline on patients' outcomes.

AGREE consists of 23 key items organised in six domains:

- **Scope and purpose** is concerned with the overall aim of the guideline, the specific clinical questions and the target patient population.
- **Stakeholder involvement** focuses on the extent to which the guideline represents the views of its intended users.
- **Rigour of development** relates to the process used to gather and synthesise the evidence and the methods used to formulate and update the recommendations.
- **Clarity and presentation** deals with the language and format of the guideline.
- **Applicability** pertains to the likely organisational, behavioural and cost implications of applying the guideline.
- **Editorial independence** is concerned with the independence of the recommendations and acknowledgement of possible conflicts of interest from the guideline development group.

Each item is rated on the extent to which a criterion has been fulfilled and scored on a four-point scale where 4 = Strongly Agree, 3 = Agree, 2 = Disagree and 1 = Strongly Disagree.

Guidelines in practice

- Clinical guidelines are not designed to replace the knowledge, skills and clinical judgement of clinicians. Guidelines need to be interpreted sensibly and applied with discretion.
- Courts are unlikely to adopt standards of care advocated in most clinical guidelines as legal 'gold standards'. The mere fact that a guideline exists does not of itself establish that compliance with it is reasonable in the circumstances or that noncompliance is negligent.

- If a guideline has been accepted by a large part of the medical profession, a clinician will need a strong reason for not following the guidance as it is likely to constitute a reasonable body of opinion for the purposes of litigation. The standards enshrined in the Bolam test may apply – minimum acceptable standards of clinical care derive from responsible customary practice[1].

1   Hurwitz B. Legal and political considerations of clinical practice guidelines. *BMJ* 1999, 318, 661–4.

SECTION E

APPLICABILITY

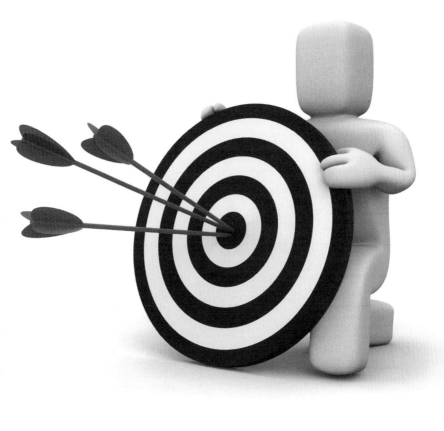

THE HIERARCHY OF EVIDENCE

There is a well-established hierarchy of research methodologies. The hierarchy is based on the premise that the study designs differ in their ability to predict what will happen to patients in real life. The studies at the top of the hierarchy carry more weight than studies lower down, because their evidence is of a higher grade.

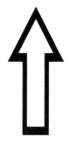

Systematic review / meta-analysis
Randomised controlled trial (RCT)
Non-randomised controlled trial
Cohort studies
Case–control studies
Cross-sectional surveys
Case series
Case report
Expert opinion
Personal communication

Studies that carry greater weight are not necessarily the best in every situation and are unlikely to be appropriate for all situations. For example, a case report can be of great importance, even though in terms of the hierarchy of studies a case report normally carries low weight. Also note that the hierarchy is for guidance only; not all studies using the same design are of equal quality.

Levels of evidence

Many organisations write systematic reviews and guidelines after reviewing the medical literature. Grading systems tend to have their foundations in the hierarchy of evidence but might be fine-tuned by giving higher scores to specific examples of good methodological practice. Ideally, grading systems should indicate the strength of the supporting evidence and the strength of the recommendation.

GRADE

Since 2000 the Grading of Recommendations Assessment, Development and Evaluation (GRADE) Working Group has developed an approach to grading quality of evidence and strength of recommendations (see www.gradeworkinggroup.org/). The overall quality of evidence is categorised as 'high', 'moderate', 'low' or 'very low'. Recommendations are only at two levels, strong or weak.

Only if clinicians are very certain that benefits do, or do not, outweigh risks and burdens on the basis of the available evidence will they make a strong recommendation. Conversely, a weak recommendation indicates that benefits and risks and burdens are finely balanced, or there is appreciable uncertainty about the magnitude of benefits and risks. A weak recommendation might also indicate that patients are liable to make different choices.

SIGN

The Scottish Intercollegiate Guidelines Network (SIGN) develops evidence-based clinical guidelines. In 2008 SIGN published *A Guideline Developer's Handbook (SIGN 50)*, which describes their approach to levels of evidence and grades of recommendation (see **Table 37**; the full document is accessible at www.sign.ac.uk/).

LEVELS OF EVIDENCE	
1++	High-quality meta-analyses, systematic reviews of RCTs, or RCTs with a very low risk of bias
1+	Well-conducted meta-analyses, systematic reviews or RCTs with a low risk of bias
1−	Meta-analyses, systematic reviews or RCTs with a high risk of bias
2++	High-quality systematic reviews of case control or cohort or studies High-quality case–control or cohort studies with a very low risk of confounding or bias and a high probability that the relationship is causal
2+	Well-conducted case–control or cohort studies with a low risk of confounding or bias and a moderate probability that the relationship is causal
2−	Case–control or cohort studies with a high risk of confounding or bias and a significant risk that the relationship is not causal
3	Non-analytic studies, eg case reports, case series
4	Expert opinion

	GRADES OF RECOMMENDATION	
A	At least one meta-analysis, systematic review or RCT rated as 1++, and directly applicable to the target population; or A body of evidence consisting principally of studies rated as 1+, directly applicable to the target population, and demonstrating overall consistency of results	
B	A body of evidence including studies rated as 2++, directly applicable to the target population, and demonstrating overall consistency of results; or Extrapolated evidence from studies rated as 1++ or 1+	
C	A body of evidence including studies rated as 2+, directly applicable to the target population and demonstrating overall consistency of results; or Extrapolated evidence from studies rated as 2++	
D	Evidence level 3 or 4; or Extrapolated evidence from studies rated as 2+	
✓	Recommended best practice based on the clinical experience of the guideline development group	

Table 37 SIGN levels of evidence and grades of recommendation. Reproduced with permission from Scottish Intercollegiate Guidelines Network.

Centre for Evidence-Based Medicine

The Oxford Centre for Evidence-Based Medicine grades the level of evidence from 1 to 5 and grades of recommendation from A to D (see the full document at www.cebm.net/index.aspx?o=5653). The Levels of Evidence table has been set out as a series of searching 'steps'. While the steps (columns) give the likely level of evidence, the level selected will also depend on (a) the nature of the question, and (b) the quality, quantity and consistency of primary evidence found at that step. Poor quality or consistency of evidence can lead to downgrading of the level; large effects or clear dose–response relationships can upgrade the level.

The final stage of critical appraisal is to determine the applicability of the research findings. By this stage you will have decided that the methodology of the study is robust and the results are significant in some way. Some research findings might be of academic interest only while others may have the potential to help your patients. Providing your patients are demographically and clinically similar to the sample population, it might be worth applying the results to your clinical practice, in the expectation that the results on your patients will be similar to the results found in the study population. One could argue that the most useful research is that which can be generalised most easily to a wider population.

Adopting an evidence-based approach to medical practice is a positive move but it is important to acknowledge that evidence-based medicine is not without its critics. The shift to statistical number crunching, the pressure to publish and the financial gains that are possible have led to abuses by doctors, researchers and marketing teams. The recommendations in a clinical paper should never be accepted at face value without considering whether a study could be accidentally or deliberately misleading.

Good critical appraisal skills will detect flaws in studies. The points listed below illustrate that the monitoring of any changes to your clinical practice is a vital step in modifying your service to an evidence-based model. If changes do not lead to improved patient care, the research should be revisited to understand why the expected benefits did not materialise.

The abstract is a summary

- The abstract is a summary of the paper, briefly describing the study's methodology, important results and key recommendations. The abstract should be considered as the sales pitch, highlighting all that is good about the paper and omitting anything bad. Abstracts are easy to read but can also mislead.

The clinical question might not be the right question

- The clinical question could have been clearly defined but might not reflect the complexity of real clinical practice. Applied in isolation, the research results might not improve practice because other important factors have not been addressed.

- Research teams composed solely of academic doctors might have priorities and viewpoints that do not reflect those of doctors at the coalface of clinical practice. Translating statistically significant results into clinical practice is not easy.

The target population is not the same as your patient population

- The target population will rarely match your patients, diminishing the generalisability of the results. The target population will be unique because of its geographical location, its culture, its morbidity and mortality levels, and differences in healthcare standards and provision.

The sample population is a sample

- The sample population is not your clinical population. It is a proportion of the target population. Whatever happens in the sample population might not happen in the target population, let alone your patients.

- People will have been excluded from the sample population but you will not be able to apply the same exclusions as easily in practice. The study results might not extrapolate to all your patients, leading to unexpected outcomes.

- People entering trials are motivated to improve their health and to follow trial protocols. They are not representative of your patients, many of whom will not meet this ideal.

- Results from small sample sizes are poor evidence for supporting big changes in clinical practice.

Randomisation might not be random

- Randomisation is vulnerable to manipulation. A poorly described allocation process, lack of robust concealment and unequal groups at baseline are warning signs that the difference between groups might have been exaggerated.

Don't be blinded by blinding

- Blinding can be compromised and almost always in favour of the researcher, improving the results because of observation bias. Open-label trials are poor evidence for change.

- Placebo preparations vary in quality. Poor matches are easily uncovered. The expectations of doctors and patients are lowered, disadvantaging those in the control arm.

- Researchers might minimise the importance of the placebo effect. Building relationships with patients and offering them hope are powerful interventions in clinical practice but are rarely discussed in research papers.

Losing subjects shows carelessness

- Results may be boosted by poor handling of subjects who withdraw or who are lost to follow-up. Every subject should be accounted for, from recruitment to outcome. Not accounting for all subjects or dismissing subjects for spurious reasons is nearly always in the researcher's favour. You will not be able to get rid of patients so easily in order to achieve comparable success rates.

Unfavourable comparisons

- Researchers sometimes compare favoured interventions with 'nobbled' comparators. Doses in the control arm might be too small for therapeutic benefit, doses might be too high and cause adverse reactions, or dosing regimens might be too onerous for subjects to follow.

- Researchers like comparing new treatments with placebo preparations but head-to-head trials with established treatments are more useful to you.

- Patients with chronic health problems are treated for months or years, yet the researchers might only provide evidence for the first few days or weeks of intervention.

- Side-effects are as important to patients as benefits but often omitted or minimised as outcome measures in research studies.

- Composite endpoints might not be valid and are difficult to translate into clinical practice and monitoring.

Statistics

- There are lies, damned lies and statistics! Data are manipulated, presented and interpreted in whichever way the researchers choose. Like a magic show, what you see is what they want you to see.

- Subgroup analyses allow researchers to focus on artificial subsets of the sample population, an exercise you will find difficult to justify to your patients.

- The focus on *P* values is unhealthy. Statistical significance is based on an arbitrary cut-off value. The magnitude of any effect should always be reported – it shows the potential impact on your patients.

- Be wary of small effect sizes, even if statistically significant. They are unlikely to benefit your patients and might not be confirmed by repeat studies.

- Small effect sizes shouldn't lead to discussions about cause and effect without a thorough examination of other factors that could play a role. Causation is usually multifactorial and not as simple as portrayed by some researchers.

- Relative risk results are less useful to you than absolute risk numbers and more likely to mislead. The impact of research is easier to exaggerate with relative risks.

- A reduction in undesirable outcomes is often presented as applying to the whole sample population whereas it only applies to those at risk. A 20% reduction in risk only applies to those who are at risk of the outcome; everyone else is unaffected. This may mean interventions are more expensive than they first appear.

The larger perspective

- Many medical breakthroughs and discoveries did not come from research trials. To practise only evidence-based medicine is to miss or ignore opportunities for improving the care of your patients.

- Statistical results apply to groups, not to individuals. Medical care should also be patient-centred, not just population-centred. Evidence-based medicine can impair the doctor–patient relationship.

- Clinical trials and marketing often overlap and can be difficult to separate. Did the clinical trial lead to the marketing campaign or did the intended marketing approach impact on the clinical trial design?

- Positive trials are much more likely to get published than negative trials. Is your impression of research skewed by publication bias? You don't know what you don't know.

CRITICAL APPRAISAL IN PRACTICE

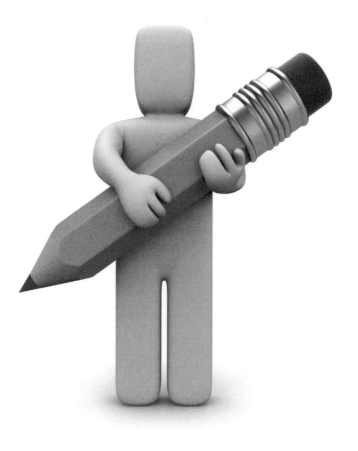

Databases

There are many different databases that cover health and medical subject areas and index research and/or high-quality information resources.

MEDLINE is produced by the National Library of Medicine in the United States (www.nlm.nih.gov). It is a major source of biomedical information and includes citations to articles from more than 4000 journals. It contains over 12 million citations dating back to the mid 1960s from international biomedical literature on all aspects of medicine and healthcare. It contains records of journal articles, bibliographic details of systematic reviews, randomised controlled trials and guidelines. There are many organisations that offer access to MEDLINE, with different ways of searching. The key MEDLINE service is offered by the US National Library of Medicine itself, in their PubMed service (www.pubmed.gov).

Cumulative Index to Nursing and Allied Health Literature (CINAHL) is a nursing and allied health database and covers topics such as health education, physiotherapy, occupational therapy, emergency services and social services in healthcare (www.ebscohost.com/cinahl). Coverage is from 1982 to the present and it is updated bimonthly.

EMBASE is the European equivalent of MEDLINE, the *Excerpta Medica* database, and is published by Elsevier Science (www.embase.com). It focuses mainly on drugs and biomedical literature and also covers health policy, drug and alcohol dependence, psychiatry, forensic science and pollution control. It covers more than 3500 journals from 110 countries and includes data from 1974 onwards. The search engine at www.embase.com includes EMBASE and unique MEDLINE records.

MEDLINE, CINAHL and EMBASE are well-established, comprehensive databases and possess sophisticated search facilities. The size of these databases requires that the searcher first defines the search terms and then refines them to reduce the number of results. Although this can be done by limiting the search by publication date, language or 'review articles only' (for example), a more valid way of limiting results is to focus on those articles that are more likely to be of high quality. This is done by using 'filters'.

NHS Economic Evaluations Database (NHS EED) is a database that focuses on economic evaluations of healthcare interventions. Economic evaluations are appraised for their quality, strengths and weaknesses. NHS EED is available from the website of the Centre for Reviews and Dissemination (www.crd.york.ac.uk/crdweb), via the Cochrane Library, via TRIP (see below) and via National electronic Library for Health (NeLH).

The **Turning Research Into Practice (TRIP)** database is a meta-search engine that searches across 61 sites of high-quality information (www.tripdatabase.com). Evidence-based publications are searched monthly by experts and indexed fully before being presented in an easy-to-use format with access to full-text articles, medical images and patient leaflets.

Intute, formerly Organising Medical Networked Information (OMNI), is a gateway to hand-selected and evaluated internet resources in health and medicine. It was created by a core team based at the University of Nottingham (access at www.intute.ac.uk).

APA PsycNET allows users to search **PsycInfo**, an abstract database of psychology literature from the 1800s to the present (http://psycnet.apa.org/). It covers more than 2000 titles, of which 98% are peer-reviewed.

Ovid HealthSTAR contains citations to the published literature on health services, technology, administration and research. It focuses on both the clinical and non-clinical aspects of healthcare delivery.

The **British Nursing Index (BNI)** indexes citations from British and English-language nursing-related journals (www.bni.org.uk).

System for Information on Grey Literature in Europe (SIGLE) is a bibliographic database covering non-conventional literature. This database is no longer being updated (www.opengrey.eu).

Google Scholar is a service from the Google search engine (http://scholar.google.com). It provides the ability to search for academic literature located across the worldwide web, including peer-reviewed papers, theses, books, abstracts and articles, from academic publishers, professional societies, preprint repositories, universities and other scholarly organisations. Google has worked with leading publishers to gain access to material that wouldn't ordinarily be accessible to search engines because it is locked behind subscription barriers. This allows users of Google Scholar to locate material of interest that would not normally be available to them. Google Scholar even attempts to rank results in order of importance.

Evidence-based medicine resources

Several journals, bulletins and newsletters cover evidence-based medicine and clinical effectiveness. Some evidence-based journals, such as the **ACP Journal Club** (www.acpjc.org), published bimonthly by the American College of Physicians, and **Evidence-Based Medicine** (http://ebm.bmjjournals. com) scrutinise articles and summarise the studies in structured abstracts, with a commentary added by a clinical expert. These journals cover reviews and choose articles that meet strict selection criteria. **Best Evidence** is a CD-ROM that contains the full text of *ACP Journal Club* and *Evidence-Based Medicine*.

Other examples of newsletters and bulletins include the **Effective Health Care** bulletins (published until 2004, www.york.ac.uk/inst/crd/ehcb.htm) and **Bandolier** (www.medicine.ox.ac.uk/bandolier/). The latter keeps doctors up to date with literature on the effectiveness of healthcare interventions.

Clinical Evidence (www.clinicalevidence.com) is a regularly updated guide to best available evidence for effective healthcare. It is a database of hundreds of clinical questions and answers and is designed to help doctors make evidence-based medicine part of their everyday practice. Topics are selected to cover important clinical conditions seen in primary care or ambulatory settings. There is rigorous peer review of all material by experts, to ensure that the information is of the highest quality. It is updated and expanded every 6 months and is published jointly by BMJ Journals and the American College of Physicians.

Evidence-Based Medicine Reviews (EBMR) is an electronic information resource that is available both via Ovid Online (www.ovid.com) and on CD-ROM. This database combines seven evidence-based medicine resources into a single searchable database: the Cochrane Collaboration's Cochrane Database of Systematic Reviews (CDSR), the Database of Abstracts of Reviews of Effectiveness (DARE), Health Technology Assessments (HTA), NHS Economic Evaluation Database (NHSEED), ACP Journal Club, the Cochrane Central Register of Controlled Trials and the Cochrane Methodology Register (CMR).

The Cochrane Collaboration

The *Cochrane Library* (www.cochrane.org) is an electronic publication designed to supply high-quality evidence to inform people providing and receiving care, and those responsible for research, teaching, funding and administration at all levels. It is a database of the Cochrane Collaboration, an international network of individuals committed to 'preparing, maintaining and promoting the accessibility of systematic reviews of the effects of healthcare'.

Development and dissemination of guidelines

The **National Library for Health (NLH)** (http://www.library.nhs.uk) provides clinicians with access to the best current know-how and knowledge to support healthcare-related decisions.

The **National Institute for Health and Clinical Excellence (NICE)** was set up as a Special Health Authority for England and Wales on 1 April 1999. It is part of the NHS and it is responsible for providing national guidance on the promotion of good health and the prevention and treatment of ill health (www.nice.org.uk).

The **NHS Centre for Reviews and Dissemination (CRD)** is based at the University of York and produces: *Effective Health Care* bulletins (systematic reviews and synthesis of research on cost- and clinical effectiveness); *Effectiveness Matters* bulletins (summaries of systematic reviews); and *Systematic Reviews of Research Evidence* (CRD reports).

The **Scottish Intercollegiate Guidelines Network (SIGN)** was formed in 1993 and its objective is to improve the effectiveness and efficiency of clinical care for patients in Scotland by developing, publishing and disseminating guidelines that identify and promote good clinical practice (www.sign.ac.uk).

The **National Guideline Clearinghouse (NGC)** is a US-based public resource for evidence-based clinical practice (www.guideline.gov).

Other sources of information

Conference proceedings: Papers given at conferences can provide important information on new research that is either in progress or recently completed. Some trials are only ever reported in conference proceedings. Databases such as the **Conference Papers Index** (www.csa.com) hold records and/or abstracts of some proceedings.

Grey literature: This is material that is not published in the standard book or journal formats. It includes reports, booklets, technical reports, circulars, newsletters and discussion papers.

Citation searching: This involves using reference lists of articles already retrieved or citation indices to trace other useful studies. The **Science Citation Index** (http://scientific.thomson.com/products/sci) allows searching for references using cited authors' surnames.

Hand searching: Journals can be physically examined for their contents. This is time-consuming, but might be a viable proposition when the published data on a topic concentrate around a few key journals.

PRESENTING AT A JOURNAL CLUB

Journal clubs are a routine fixture in academic programmes at teaching hospitals. A successful presentation requires preparation, good presentation skills and clinical relevance for the audience.

Preparation

Different journal clubs take different approaches to the running of the meetings. Some journal clubs are very prescriptive – the clinical paper is already chosen and the doctor has to simply appraise it. Other clubs rely on the doctor to choose a paper of his or her choice. Some clubs ask the doctor to search for and appraise a paper related to a clinical question of interest, such as a question raised by a recent case presentation. However the clinical paper is chosen, preparation has to start well in advance of the presentation.

Ideally, you should distribute the clinical paper to the journal club members at least a week in advance. Most articles are available to download as Adobe Acrobat files from the journal websites; this format maintains their original formatting and provides an excellent original for photocopying. However, be aware of copyright restrictions on distribution. An alternative approach is to publicise the link to the article on the World Wide Web. When you distribute information about your chosen paper, include information on the timing of the journal club and intimate that you will expect everyone to have read the paper before the presentation, which will focus on the critical appraisal of it.

Presentation skills

Nowadays it is not excusable to use anything less than an LCD projector with Microsoft PowerPoint or an equivalent software package for your presentation.

Using PowerPoint

PowerPoint makes it easy to produce great-looking presentations, but its flexibility and ease of use also allow doctors to produce presentations that look anything but professional. Use its template features to give your presentation a consistent and professional appearance. Journal clubs are formal affairs, so stick to a dark background colour for your slides, such as blue or black, with lightly coloured text to keep the presentation sober-looking and to aid readability. Avoid patterned backgrounds and fussy templates, which will distract the audience from your presentation. Use a traditional serif typeface, such as

Times New Roman, and avoid typefaces that give an informal impression or try to mimic handwriting.

Slide content

Keep each slide brief and to the point. Every slide should have a title and up to five bullet points, on which you will expand during the presentation. Consider using tables or diagrams to summarise information. Avoid abbreviations and acronyms in your presentation, unless your audience is familiar with them. Make sure you double-check your spelling and grammar. Pay particular attention to the appropriate use of capital letters and punctuation marks. Avoid fancy slide transitions, animations and sound effects.

Delivering the slide show

Dress smartly for your presentation. Leave your mobile phone or pager with a colleague. Arrive early at the journal club, set up your presentation and make sure all the slides appear as designed – don't expect that the technology will always work.

During the presentation, stand to one side of the screen. Talk clearly to the audience, and not too quickly. Make eye contact with different members of the audience for a few seconds at a time. Wireless remote controls, such as the Logitech Cordless Presenter with its built-in timer and laser pointer, enable you to advance through your slides without having to use the keyboard or stand next to the computer. Using such a device can be a liberating experience.

Slides

The organisation of the slides depends on the subject matter. Below is an example of a slide presentation. Resist the temptation to simply read out an abbreviated form of the research paper – your audience has already read it!

SLIDE 1	SLIDE 2
The title of the paper The author(s) of the paper Journal name and date of publication Your name and other details	The clinical question the paper aims to answer The primary hypothesis Comment on the background to this project Comment on originality

SLIDE 3	SLIDE 4
The study design – is it appropriate?	The target population Inclusion and exclusion criteria The sample population The sample size and power calculations

SLIDE 5	SLIDE 6
The randomisation process Concealed allocation	Interventions The blinding process Bias and confounding factors identified

SLIDE 7	SLIDE 8
The outcome measures Validity and reliability of measurements	The null hypothesis Describe the main results

SLIDE 9	SLIDE 10
The statistical methods used Intention-to-treat analysis Completeness of follow-up	Were the aims of the study fulfilled? Are the relevant findings justified? Are the conclusions of the paper justified?

SLIDE 11	SLIDE 12
What is the impact of the paper? Can the results be generalised to your hospital's population?	What do you think of the paper? Summarise the good and bad points What future work can be done? Any questions?

TAKING PART IN AN AUDIT MEETING

The word 'audit' is guaranteed to divide doctors into two camps. On one side are those doctors who leap at the opportunity to improve the services they offer patients. On the other side are those doctors who detest the idea that they should be taken away from clinical work to engage in what they perceive to be a managerial duty. Whatever their attitude to audit is, however, most doctors find themselves doing audits because career progression often depends on being able to show evidence of completed audit projects. Importantly, successful audit outcomes depend on a multidisciplinary team approach to ensure practical and timely interventions to improve services. Doctors not engaging in audit do so at their peril and to the detriment of the service as a whole.

Audit meetings usually take place regularly on a monthly basis. To maintain audience interest and continuity, each audit meeting should have on its agenda a mixture of audit presentations, audit protocols for approval and an opportunity for members of the audience to propose audit titles. A rolling agenda should be kept to ensure that teams present their audit projects at the proposal and protocol stages as well as at the end of the first and second cycles of data collection. Only then will audit projects be completed and make a meaningful difference to service provision. Unfortunately it is all too common to see audit projects abandoned after the first data collection as a result of apathy, doctors moving to different hospitals or a poor understanding of the audit cycle. Each project should have an audit lead who will see the project through to its conclusion.

It is important to distinguish between audits, surveys and research projects. Far too often, surveys of service provision are presented as audits where there is no intention of comparing the findings with a gold standard or repeating the data collection after putting an intervention in place. Other doctors present research projects as audits as a way of sidestepping ethics committees because audit projects do not normally require ethics approval. The chair of the audit meeting needs to keep the meeting focused on audit projects and nothing else.

Opposite is an example of a slide presentation of an audit protocol. Discussions after such presentations tend to focus on the details of the gold standard of service provision with which the local service will be compared. It is imperative that research is done prior to selecting the gold standard to ensure that it is the gold standard! This can mean seeking out national as well as local guidelines on best practice. In the absence of a recognised gold standard, the team might need to make one up or follow the advice of a key opinion leader.

SLIDE 1	SLIDE 2
The title of the audit project The names of the audit lead and participants Date of presentation	A description of the aspect of the service that might need to be improved

SLIDE 3	SLIDE 4
The gold standard for that part of the service	Details of the first cycle of data collection Who will collect the data and when? What data will be collected?

SLIDE 5	SLIDE 6
The audit tool in more detail	Date of presentation of first data collection and comparison with the gold standard Any questions?

The audit tool is an instrument that facilitates the data collection and this can be done on a retrospective or prospective basis. It is usually a blank form to be filled in with data. The audit tool should be designed to collect only meaningful data and not be overinclusive. The simpler the audit project, the more likely it is to be completed!

After the first collection of data, the comparison of the local service with the gold standard should be presented at the audit meeting. At this point possible interventions to bring the standard of the local service closer to the gold standard should be discussed with the audience. As far as possible the selected interventions should be pragmatic, likely to succeed and incorporate fail-safe methods.

The completion of the audit cycle requires a final presentation on the second collection of data after the implementation of the agreed interventions. There is, however, no limit to the number of times any aspect of the service can be re-audited.

Done well, audit projects can lead to healthcare environments and procedures that are better suited to the needs of both doctors and patients. It is unlikely that any doctor would complain about that!

WORKING WITH PHARMACEUTICAL REPRESENTATIVES

Doctors differ in their attitudes towards the pharmaceutical industry.

Without a doubt, pharmaceutical companies have revolutionised the practice of medicine. They have invested tremendous amounts in research activity to bring products to the marketplace that benefit our patients. Without their financial clout, many products would simply never have been in a position to be licensed.

The reputation of some pharmaceutical companies has been tarnished in recent years, however, because of the conflict between their research and marketing departments. The companies exist, after all, to sell products and generate profits. However, as doctors, we should be able to focus our attention on the research work, so that we can decide whether or not our clinical practice can be improved.

The company representative role has evolved over the years in recognition of the changes in the NHS and the acceptance of an evidence-based approach to treatments. In addition to representatives who focus purely on sales in primary and/or secondary care, there are representatives who work on NHS issues with commissioners and, in some companies, staff who work with outcomes research. Different representatives' objectives will not be the same! An understanding of the roles and responsibilities of pharmaceutical representatives will enable you to maximise the benefits of meeting with them regularly.

The sales representative dissected

Before meeting with you, a pharmaceutical sales representative will know a lot about you. Information about your prescribing habits will have been gleaned from data on dispensed prescriptions. The representative wants to meet you because you are in a position to increase the sales of their company's products. This might be accomplished by issuing more prescriptions, by advocating the use of their products to other prescribers, or because you are involved in research that could be favourable to their products.

After the usual greetings and niceties, the focus of the discussion will move to your prescribing habits. The representative wants to gain an insight into how you make decisions about prescribing issues. This involves asking questions about the types of patients you see, the products you prescribe, the reasons for your choice of first-line medications and your experiences with and prejudices against alternative approaches.

The representative will assess your needs in terms of identifying groups of patients in which your outcomes could be improved. They will talk about their company's products and show you evidence of the benefits of prescribing these products for your patients. Sales aids, PowerPoint presentations, promotional literature and clinical papers will magically appear from black briefcases. The effect can be overwhelming, as you are blinded by volumes of impressive data. The representative finishes off the presentation and questioning and asks for some commitment in terms of trying the company's product.

The doctor's viewpoint

Being a passive observer in a meeting with a sales representative is not a good use of your time. The representative is usually very knowledgeable about his or her specialist field and is a potential source of a lot of useful information. You will have your own needs in terms of information you need in order to be a better doctor, and by identifying these needs to the representative, you can both be in a win–win situation.

There are general questions you can ask to update your knowledge base:

- What is the latest research the company is doing?
- Are there any impending licence changes or new launches?
- Are there any forthcoming NHS initiatives that I should be aware of?
- Which guidelines are in vogue, and who are the key opinion leaders?

If the representative is selling a product to you, you need to focus the discussion on information that will help you to decide whether or not to prescribe the product. Questions you might ask about the data presented can include the following:

- Are these efficacy data or effectiveness data?
- Is the sample population similar to our own?
- What were the inclusion and exclusion criteria?
- What was the comparative treatment? Was it a placebo or was it a head-to-head trial?
- Do the doses used in the study reflect everyday clinical practice?
- What was the absolute risk reduction with the new treatment?

- What was the number needed to treat?
- Are the results statistically significant and clinically significant?
- In which situations should the new treatment not be prescribed?
- Are there any safety data we need to be aware of?
- Why should we not prescribe a competitor product?
- Is this a cost-effective intervention?
- Are there any post-marketing studies in progress?
- Has the drug been through the Drugs and Therapeutics Committee, or has a pharmaceutical advisor been presented with the data?

If you are presented with any graphs, put your analytical skills to the test by looking for marketing tricks in the presentation of data. Examples include magnification of the Y axis to exaggerate differences in comparative results, and poor labelling of the X axis in an attempt to hide the short duration of a trial.

Sources of information

Promotional material
The representative can give you approved promotional materials that list product features and benefits. Sales aids help convey important information such as data on efficacy, safety, tolerability, compliance, comparative data with competitors, health-economic data, the summary of product characteristics and the price.

Clinical papers
Clinical papers provide you with the original data on which promotional material is based. If you prefer to look at the clinical papers, ask the representative to go through the relevant papers or, alternatively, ask for copies to be sent to you. Once you have the paper, you will want to appraise it critically yourself and then arrange to meet with the representative to discuss any issues or questions that you have. An experienced representative will be able to critique the paper as they use it to sell to you, and point out key details.

Key opinion leaders
You might want to know the opinion of specialists in a field before you prescribe a certain drug. Ask your representative about key opinion leaders and whether they can arrange for you to meet with these people or hear them speak at an appropriate scientific meeting. Alternatively, ask to set up a round-table meeting with you and your colleagues so that you can have an open discussion with the

expert about the product and how it would benefit your patients. If you would like to be an advocate for the product, then tell the representative to arrange meetings for you to discuss this with your colleagues.

Data on file

If there is information presented that you are interested in but which has not yet been published, it is usually referenced as 'data on file'. If you would like to see these data, you can request the information and the representative will contact their medical department, who will send this on to you.

Off-licence data

If you have queries that are off-licence, you should let the representative know. They will contact their medical department, and either someone from that department will come to see you or they will send you the requested information. The representative is not allowed to discuss off-licence information.

FURTHER READING

The *JAMA* series

1. Guyatt GH, Sackett DL, Cook DJ, for the Evidence-Based Medicine Working Group. Users' guides to the medical literature. II. How to use an article about therapy or prevention. A. Are the results of the study valid? *Journal of the American Medical Association* 1993, 270, 2598–601.

2. Guyatt GH, Sackett DL, Cook DJ, for the Evidence-Based Medicine Working Group. Users' guides to the medical literature. II. How to use an article about therapy or prevention. B. What were the results and will they help me in caring for my patients? *Journal of the American Medical Association* 1994, 271, 59–63.

3. Jaeschke R, Guyatt G, Sackett DL. Users' guides to the medical literature. III. How to use an article about a diagnostic test. A. Are the results of the study valid? *Journal of the American Medical Association* 1994, 271, 389–91.

4. Jaeschke R, Gordon H, Guyatt G, Sackett DL, for the Evidence-Based Medicine Working Group. Users' guides to the medical literature. III. How to use an article about a diagnostic test. B. What are the results and will they help me in caring for my patients? *Journal of the American Medical Association* 1994, 271, 703–7.

5. Levine M, Walter S, Lee H, et al., for the Evidence-Based Medicine Working Group. Users'guides to the medical literature. IV. How to use an article about harm. *Journal of the American Medical Association* 1994, 271, 1615–19.

6. Laupacis A, Wells G, Richardson S, Tugwell P, for the Evidence-Based Medicine Working Group. Users' guides to the medical literature. V. How to use an article about prognosis. *Journal of the American Medical Association* 1994, 272, 234–7.

7. Oxman AD, Cook DJ, Guyatt GH, for the Evidence-Based Medicine Working Group. Users' guides to the medical literature. VI. How to use an overview. *Journal of the American Medical Association* 1994, 272, 1367–71.

8. Drummond MF, Richardson WS, O'Brien BJ, Levine M, Heyland D, for the Evidence-Based Medicine Working Group. Users' guides to the medical literature. XIII. How to use an article on economic analysis of clinical practice. A. Are the results of the study valid? *Journal of the American Medical Association* 1997, 277, 1552–7.

9. O'Brien BJ, Heyland D, Richardson WS, Levine M, Drummond MF, for the Evidence-Based Medicine Working Group. Users' guides to the medical literature. XIII. How to use an article on economic analysis of clinical practice. B. What are the results and will they help me in caring for my patients? *Journal of the American Medical Association* 1997, 277, 1802–6. Published erratum appears in *JAMA* 1997, 278, 1064.

10. Barratt A, Irwig L, Glasziou P, et al., for the Evidence-Based Medicine Working Group. Users' guide to medical literature. XVII. How to use guidelines and recommendations about screening. *Journal of the American Medical Association* 1999, 281, 2029–34.

11. Giacomini MK, Cook DJ, for the Evidence-Based Medicine Working Group. Users' guides to the medical literature. XXIII. Qualitative research in health care. A. Are the results of the study valid? *Journal of the American Medical Association* 2000, 284, 357–62.

12. Giacomini MK, Cook DJ, for the Evidence-Based Medicine Working Group. Users' guides to the medical literature. XXIII. Qualitative research in health care. B. What are the results and how do they help me care for my patients? *Journal of the American Medical Association* 2000, 284, 478–82.

The 'How to read a paper' series

A readable and practical series, originally published in the *BMJ*.

1. Greenhalgh T. How to read a paper: the Medline database. *BMJ* 1997, 315, 180–3.

2. Greenhalgh T. How to read a paper: getting your bearings (deciding what the paper is about). *BMJ* 1997, 315, 243–6.

3. Greenhalgh T. How to read a paper: assessing the methodological quality of published papers. *BMJ* 1997, 315, 305–8.

4. Greenhalgh T. How to read a paper: statistics for the non-statistician. I: Different types of data need different statistical tests. *BMJ* 1997, 315, 364–6.

5. Greenhalgh T. How to read a paper: statistics for the non-statistician. II: 'Significant' relations and their pitfalls. *BMJ* 1997, 315, 422–5.

6. Greenhalgh T. How to read a paper: papers that report drug trials. *BMJ* 1997, 315, 480–3.

7. Greenhalgh T. How to read a paper: papers that report diagnostic or screening tests. *BMJ* 1997, 315, 540–3.

8. Greenhalgh T. How to read a paper: papers that tell you what things cost (economic analyses). *BMJ* 1997, 315, 596–9.

9. Greenhalgh T. How to read a paper: papers that summarise other papers (systematic reviews and meta-analyses). *BMJ* 1997, 315, 672–5.

10. Greenhalgh T. How to read a paper: papers that go beyond numbers (qualitative research). *BMJ* 1997, 315, 740–3.

Other useful online resources

The **Critical Appraisal Skills Programme (CASP)** is part of the Public Health Resource Unit based at Oxford (www.phru.nhs.uk/Pages/PHD/CASP. htm). CASP runs training workshops on critical appraisal skills. This site also contains some of their checklists for appraising research.

The **Evidence-Based Medicine Toolkit** is hosted by the University of Alberta (www.ebm.med.ualberta.ca). It is an online 'box' of handy tools to help you find, appraise and apply evidence-based research.

Levels of Evidence and Grades of Recommendation is a ranking system used to rank various study designs in order of evidence-based merit (www.cebm.net/levels_of_evidence.asp). Systematic reviews or meta-analyses and well-conducted randomised controlled trials are usually seen as the best form of 'evidence', with research based on the outcome of a case series placed somewhere near the bottom.

The Trent Research and Development Support Unit Research Information Access Gateway (TRIAGE) is a very good list of links to critical appraisal resources compiled by the School of Health and Related Research (ScHARR) at Sheffield (www.trentrdsu.org.uk/resources.html). The TRIAGE site provides links to teaching materials, tutorials and articles related to all areas of health research and evidence-based medicine.

Self-assessment exercise 1

Any other significant findings should be regarded as exploratory only, and perhaps give you ideas for further research projects.

Self-assessment exercise 2

1. Case–control study
2. Cohort study
3. Audit
4. Randomised controlled trial
5. Qualitative study
6. Economic analysis

Self-assessment exercise 3

1. All your patients are given the gold-standard test for meningitis – lumbar puncture. They are also given the blood test that you have developed. The results from the new test are compared with those of the gold-standard test.

2. Your patients will be randomly allocated to one of two groups. One group will receive the new treatment. The other group will receive either a placebo treatment or a pre-existing treatment. After a period of time the results of the two interventions will be compared.

3. You could choose a case–control study, looking at the risk factors to which patients with and without schizophrenia have been exposed in the past. Alternatively, you could choose a cohort study design, following up people who smoke / don't smoke cannabis to see if they develop schizophrenia.

4. A cohort study of people with and without frozen shoulder, where subjects are followed up to see if they return to work. Alternatively, one could look at people working and not working and see how many of them have been diagnosed with frozen shoulder.

Self-assessment exercise 4

1. A crossover design requires fewer subjects than a randomised controlled trial because the subjects are their own controls, so they are matched with themselves. However, crossover designs suffer with order effects, historical controls and carry-over effects.

2. Cohort studies observe people who have been exposed to a risk factor to see if they develop an outcome. Case–control studies look at people who already have the outcome and investigate what risk factors they have been exposed to in the past. For investigating rare exposures, cohort studies are better. For investigating rare outcomes, case–control studies are preferred.

3. As a clinician, you should only audit aspects of the service in which you are involved. For example, if you are a doctor in a hospital setting, you should not audit aspects of service provision in a primary-care setting. If you did want to audit something that is related to your service but is managed in the primary-care setting, it would be acceptable to do a joint project with a colleague who is working in primary care.

Self-assessment exercise 5

1. Selection bias: Patients who have suffered cerebrovascular accidents might no longer live at home or they might be unable to answer the phone.

2. Observation bias: Teenagers might be reluctant to answer questions about drug misuse if questioned by a figure of authority.

3. Selection bias: There will be a concentration of such cases on the ward, resulting in a stronger association than perhaps there is in reality.

4. Observation bias: In the glow of motherhood or after the trauma of childbirth, women might not accurately recall the pain of delivery and the interventions used.

Self-assessment exercise 6

1. Smoking cigarettes
2. Fair skin
3. Smoking
4. Poverty

Self-assessment exercise 7

Inclusion criteria include:

- Adult age group 18–65 years (licence restrictions; criteria for admission to adult wards)
- Diagnosed with schizoaffective disorder
- Hospital inpatient

Exclusion criteria include:

- Already taking risperidone
- Treatment failure with risperidone in the past (ethical consideration)
- Comorbid medical and psychiatric conditions
- Coexisting alcohol or drug misuse
- Unable to give informed consent

Self-assessment exercise 8

1. Annual incidence rate of lung cancer in the exposed group

 = 4 cases in 100 men in 10 years
 = 0.4 cases in 100 men in 1 year
 = 0.4% annual incidence rate

Annual incidence rate in unexposed group

 = 1 case in 100 men in 10 years
 = 0.1 case in 100 men in 1 year
 = 0.1% annual incidence rate

Overall incidence rate

 = 5 cases in 200 men in 10 years
 = 0.5 cases in 200 men in 1 year
 = 0.25 cases in 100 men in 1 year
 = 0.25% annual incidence rate

2. 90 babies delivered every month

= 1080 babies delivered every year
1 in 2500 babies affected by cystic fibrosis, ie 0.04%
0.04% of 1080 = 0.432 babies every year = about 4 babies every 10 years

3. 1.3 people in every 100 000 die each year from pancreatitis
= 780 people in every 60 million die each year from pancreatitis
= 15 people in every 60 million die each week from pancreatitis

4. 85 000 people with multiple sclerosis in a population of 60 million
= 141 people with multiple sclerosis in a population of 100 000
prevalence rate = 141 per 100 000

5. Effects on prevalence:

    a. Increased
    b. Decreased
    c. Decreased
    d. Decreased

Self-assessment exercise 9

1. $\text{risk} = \dfrac{10}{60} = 0.166 = 16.6\%$

   $\text{odds} = \dfrac{10}{50} = 0.2$

2. 5% of 220 = 11

3.

		LUNG DISEASE		
		yes	no	Totals
EXPOSURE TO ASBESTOS	positive	20	36	56
	negative	2	42	44
Totals		22	78	100

$\text{CER} = \dfrac{2}{44} = 4.5\%$

$$EER = \frac{20}{56} = 35.7\%$$

$$\text{Odds in exposed group} = \frac{20}{36} = 0.56$$

$$\text{Odds in non-exposed group} = \frac{2}{42} = 0.05$$

4.

		FUNGAL NAIL INFECTION		
		yes	no	Totals
GIVEN NEW TREATMENT	positive	21	979	1000
	negative	66	934	1000
Totals		87	1913	2000

$$\text{Absolute risk in the treated group (EER)} = \frac{21}{1000} = 0.021 = 2.1\%$$

$$\text{Absolute risk in the untreated group (CER)} = \frac{66}{1000} = 0.066 = 6.6\%$$

$$\text{Relative risk} = \frac{0.021}{0.066} = 0.32 = 32\% \text{ (an improvement)}$$

$$\text{Relative risk reduction} = \frac{0.066 - 0.021}{0.066} = 0.68$$

$$\text{Absolute risk reduction} = 0.066 - 0.021 = 0.045$$

$$\text{The number needed to treat} = \frac{1}{0.045} = 22$$

5.

		PAIN SYMPTOMS		
		yes	no	Totals
GIVEN NEW ANALGESIC	positive	4	17	21
	negative	19	1	20
Totals		23	18	41

$$CER = \frac{19}{20} = 0.95$$

$$EER = \frac{4}{21} = 0.19$$

Odds ratio = 4 × 1 / 17 × 19 = 0.012

Self-assessment exercise 10

1.
   a. Qualitative, nominal
   b. Qualitative, nominal
   c. Quantitative, continuous, ratio
   d. Qualitative, ordinal
   e. Quantitative, continuous, ratio
   f. Qualitative, nominal
   g. Quantitative, continuous, ratio
   h. Qualitative, nominal
   i. Quantitative, continuous, interval
   j. Qualitative, nominal
   k. Qualitative, ordinal

Self-assessment exercise 11

1.

    a.   mode = 3

    b.   frequencies: value 1 (1), value 2 (2), value 3 (3), value 4 (2), value 5 (1)

    c.   median = 3

    d.   range = 5 − 1 = 4

    e.   mean $= \dfrac{1 + 2 + 2 + 3 + 3 + 3 + 4 + 4 + 5}{9} = 3$

2.

    a.

       median = 15

    b.   range = 100 − 5 = 95

    c.   mean $= \dfrac{5 + 10 + 15 + 20 + 100}{5} = 30$

    d.   The median describes the central tendency of this data set better because it is less affected by outlying values

3.

    a.   median $= \dfrac{30 + 35}{2} = 32.5$

    b.   range = 70 − 5 = 65

    c.   interquartile range

    i.   split data into quarters: 5, 10, 15 | 20, 25, 30 | 35, 40, 45 | 50, 60, 70

    ii.   1st quartile lies between 15 and 20 = 17.5

    iii.   3rd quartile lies between 45 and 50 = 47.5

    iv.   interquartile range = 47.5 − 17.5 = 30

4.

    a.   mean $= \dfrac{3 + 13 + 44 + 45 + 51 + 56 + 66 + 75 + 91 + 102}{10}$

       $= 54.6$

    b.   standard deviation $= \sqrt{\dfrac{(x - \bar{x})^2}{n - 1}}$

Calculate $(x - \bar{x})^2$ for all the values

$(3 - 54.6)^2 = 2662.56$

$(13 - 54.6)^2 = 1730.56$

$(44 - 54.6)^2 = 112.36$

$(45 - 54.6)^2 = 92.16$

$(51 - 54.6)^2 = 12.96$

$(56 - 54.6)^2 = 1.96$

$(66 - 54.6)^2 = 129.96$

$(75 - 54.6)^2 = 416.16$

$(91 - 54.6)^2 = 1324.96$

$(102 - 54.6)^2 = 2246.76$

Add all the $(x - \bar{x})^2$ values   8730.4

Divide by $n - 1$ ($n = 10$) $\dfrac{8730.4}{10 - 1}$ = 970.04

Standard deviation is the square root of the result $\sqrt{970.04}$ = 31.15

c. 95% of observations will lie within 2 standard deviations on either side of the mean:

mean = 54.6

standard deviation = 31.15

2 standard deviations = $31.15 \times 2 = 62.3$

range = $54.6 \pm 62.3 = -7.7$ to 116.9

Self-assessment exercise 12

1.
   - a. mean = 16
   - b. median = 17
   - c. standard deviation = 3.9
   - d. standard error = 1.47

2.
   - a. mean = 26
   - b. median = 17
   - c. standard deviation = 28.8
   - d. standard error = 10.88

Self-assessment exercise 13

1. Paroxetine is not associated with discontinuation symptoms.
2. Atorvastatin is as effective at lowering cholesterol levels as simvastatin

    or

    Atorvastatin is no more effective than simvastatin at lowering cholesterol levels.

Self-assessment exercise 14

1. First draw a 2 × 2 table

		DISEASE STATUS BY GOLD STANDARD		
		positive	negative	Totals
DISEASE STATUS BY NEW TEST	positive	32	2	34
	negative	1	101	102
Totals		33	103	136

a.

$$\text{Sensitivity} = \frac{32}{33} = 0.97$$

$$\text{Specificity} = \frac{101}{103} = 0.98$$

$$\text{Positive predictive value} = \frac{32}{32 + 2} = 0.94$$

$$\text{Negative predictive value} = \frac{101}{1 + 101} = 0.99$$

b.

$$\text{Likelihood ratio for a positive test result} = \frac{0.97}{1 - 0.98} = 48.5$$

$$\text{Likelihood ratio for a negative test result} = \frac{1 - 0.97}{0.98} = 0.03$$

c.

$$\text{Pre-test probability} = \frac{32 + 1}{32 + 2 + 1 + 101} = 0.24$$

$$\text{Pre-test odds} = \frac{0.24}{1 - 0.24} = 0.31$$

$$\text{Post-test odds} = 0.31 \times 48.5 = 15.03$$

$$\text{Post-test probability} = \frac{15.03}{15.03 + 1} = 0.94$$

It is never an easy task to initiate, plan and complete a research project. It requires dedication, hard work and a willingness to work long hours, which are often unpaid and unrecognised. Few researchers aim deliberately to publish poor-quality research. More often than not, limitations in trial design and conduct are due to a lack of resources, ethical considerations or simply that pragmatic solutions have to be found to enable the research project to take place.

The attainment of critical appraisal skills allows doctors to evaluate the quality of research papers. Such skills should be used not only to find flaws in clinical papers, but also to comment positively on the good points. Taking a balanced approach will ensure that all research, good and bad, generates ideas for future projects. It is this endless cycle of thinking, questioning and doing that has brought us so far. The journey is far from complete.

In 1676, Isaac Newton wrote to a fellow scientist, acknowledging the work of others in his own research:

If I have seen further, it is by standing on the shoulders of giants.

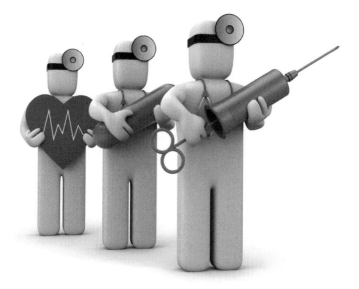

INDEX

2 x 2 tables (contingency tables) 91–4, 98–9, 130, 166
  self-assessment exercises 98–9, 224–6

a priori (primary) hypothesis 19–20
absolute risk (AR) 95
absolute risk reduction (ARR) 94, 95, 99, 225
  negative 98
abstracts 13, 198
accuracy (validity) 70, 72–3, 81, 167
adaptive randomisation 58–9
adverse drug reactions 24, 64
aetiological studies (causation) 19, 25–9, 162–3
AGREE Instrument (for guidelines) 190–1
allocation (randomisation methods) 33–4, 51, 56–61, 199
alternative hypothesis 121, 126
  see also null hypothesis
alternative-form reliability 76
analysis of variance (ANOVA) 132, 133, 135–6
AR see absolute risk
ARR see absolute risk reduction
articles
  quality assessment 11–12, 32–5, 146–7, 198–201
  structure 13–14, 17
attrition bias 45, 47, 86
audit 36–7, 212–13, 222
authors 13
average see mean; median

Bandolier website 207
baseline characteristics 42, 55
Bayes' theorem 174
bell-shaped curve 109
Berkson bias 46
Bernoulli distribution 106
Best Evidence (ACP/BMJ) 207

bias in design/execution 44–8, 188, 222
  prevention 54–61, 65–8, 86–90, 188
bias in publication 45, 155–7
binary data 100, 134, 135, 143
binomial distribution 106, 143
Bland–Altman limits of agreement 75
blinding 34, 61, 65–7, 199–200
block randomisation 57
BNI database (British Nursing Index) 206
Bonferroni correction 127
Boolean operators 9

carry-over effects 31
case–cohort studies 28
case–control studies 26–9, 55, 97, 196
  self-assessment exercises 39, 221, 222
case reports 24
case series 24
CASP (Critical Appraisal Skills Programme) 220
categorical (qualitative) data 100, 102, 103, 104, 226
  analytical statistics 129–31, 134, 135, 143
  descriptive statistics 108
  reliability 75–6
causation 28–9
causation studies (aetiological) 19, 25–8, 162–3
censored data 176, 177
censuses 37
central limit theorem 106
Centre for Evidence-Based Medicine 197
CER see control event rate
checklists 161, 218–19
  aetiological studies 163
  diagnostic studies 165, 172
  economic studies 179
  prognostic studies 175

qualitative research 186
treatment studies 173–4
chi-squared (^{2}) test 130, 152–3
CI see confidence interval
CINAHL (Current Index to Nursing and
Allied Health Literature) 205
citations 11–12, 146, 208
class effects 138
Clinical Evidence (ACP/BMJ) 207
clinical questions 7–8, 18–21, 146,
198–9
clinical significance 127
clinical trials 40–1, 196
see also study design
cluster analysis 144
cluster randomisation 23, 58
cluster sampling 43
Cochrane Collaboration 1, 150, 207
Cochran's Q 152–3
coefficient of determination (r^2) 140
coefficient of variation 75, 111
Cohen's statistic (κ) 75–6
cohort studies 25–6, 27–8, 55, 176–7
self-assessment exercises 39, 221,
222
composite endpoints 69–70
concealed allocation 60–1
concurrent validity 72
conferences 208
confidence interval (CI) 119–20, 127–8
in forest plots 148
conflicts of interest 14
confounding factors 49–53, 55, 223
consent 58
CONSORT statement 32–5
constant comparison analysis 189
construct validity 73
content analysis 189
content validity 72
contingency tables 91–4, 130, 166
self-assessment exercises 98–9,
224–6
continuous data 100–1, 102–3
analytical statistics 131–44
descriptive statistics 105, 106–7,
109–20, 227–9
reliability 75
control event rate (CER) 94, 95, 96
self-assessment exercises 98–9, 224,
225, 226

controlled trials 30
see also randomised controlled trials
convenience sampling 43
convergent validity 73
correlation 139–41
intraclass correlation coefficient 75
see also regression
cost–benefit analysis 183–4
cost–consequences analysis 182
cost-effectiveness analysis 19, 181–2
cost-minimisation analysis 181
cost-of-illness studies 180
cost–utility analysis 182–3
covariance 52, 136
Cox proportional hazards regression
144, 178
criterion validity 72–3
critical appraisal, overview 5, 198–201
Critical Appraisal Skills Programme
(CASP) 220
Crohnbach's alpha (α) 74
crossover trials 30–1, 222
cross-sectional studies 22, 37
cut-off point optimisation 171–2

data dredging 20
databases 205–6, 207
interrogation of 9–10, 146
death rates 82–3, 85, 224
degrees of freedom 131
diagnostic purity bias 46, 54
diagnostic studies 19, 164–72, 229–30
discrete data (quantitative) 100, 105,
106
distribution 105–20, 227–9
divergent validity 73
double-dummy technique 66
drop-outs (missing data) 86–90, 176,
200

ecological studies 22
economic analysis 37, 179–84, 206
EER see experimental event rate
effect size 112, 125, 152, 201
Effective Health Care bulletins 207
effectiveness 5–6, 22
efficacy 5–6, 22
EMBASE database 205
endpoints 69–77
see also missing data

epidemiological studies 82–5, 223–4
equivalence studies 137
ethics 63–4, 158
evidence-based medicine 3–10, 198,
    201, 207
    levels and grades of evidence 195–7,
    220
Evidence-Based Medicine Toolkit 220
exclusion (attrition) bias 45, 47, 86
exclusion criteria 51, 54, 223
experimental event rate (EER) 94, 95,
    96
    self-assessment exercises 98–9, 224,
    225, 226
experimental studies 30–5, 40–1,
    221–2
experts 11, 216–17

F value 174
face validity 72
factor analysis 144
factorial studies 32
false-negative results (type 2 errors) 88,
    124–6, 127
false-positive results (type 1 errors) 20,
    90, 123–4, 124–5, 127
financial (economic) analysis 37,
    179–84, 206
Fisher's exact test 130
fixed randomisation 57–8
fixed-effects model 152
focus groups 187
forest plots 148–9, 152
frequency 108, 116, 227
Friedman's test 132
funnel plots 155–7

Galbraith plots 153
Gaussian (normal) distribution 106–7,
    109–12, 133
geometric mean 113–14
Google Scholar 206
GRADE (Grading of Recommendations
    Assessment, Development and
    Evaluation) 195–6
grey literature 146, 206, 208
grounded theory 186
guidelines 150, 190–2, 208

hand searching 146, 208

Hawthorne effect 47
hazard rate/ratio 144, 178
heterogeneity of study results 151–4
hierarchy of evidence 195–7, 220
historical control bias 46
hospital standardised mortality ratio 83
'How to read a paper' series 219–20
hypotheses
    null/alternative 121–8, 229
    primary/secondary 19–20

I-squared statistic 153
immediacy index 12
imputation 87
inception cohorts 26
incidence 83–4, 85, 223–4
inclusion criteria 51, 54, 223
incremental validity 73
infectious diseases 29
information sources 150, 205–8,
    218–20
intention-to-treat analysis 86–90
interim analysis 158
internet resources 12, 150, 205–8, 220
    search strategies 9–10, 146
interquartile range 114–15, 116, 227
inter-rater reliability 74, 75–6
interval scales 102, 103, 134
interviewer bias 47
interviews, in qualitative research 188
intraclass correlation coefficient 75
intrarater reliability 74
Intute website 206

Journal of the American Medical
    Association (JAMA) 218–19
journal clubs 209–11
journal impact factor 12
journals
    databases 9–10, 205–7
    relative quality of 11–12
    see also articles

Kaplan–Meier survival analysis 176–7
kappa statistic (κ) 75–6
Kendall's correlation coefficient (τ) 141
Koch's postulates 29
Kruskal–Wallis ANOVA test 132
kurtosis 115

L'Abbé plots 153
'last observation carried forward' method 87, 88–90
least squares method 143
legal status of guidelines 191–2
likelihood ratio 167, 169–70, 172, 230
linear regression 52–3, 142–3
literature review 9–12, 146
log–rank test 178
log transformation of data 113–14, 120
logistic regression 52, 143
longitudinal studies 22, 176–7

Mann–Whitney U test 132
MANOVA/MANCOVA (multiple analysis of [co]variance) 136
Mantel–Haenszel procedure 52, 152
manual searching 146, 208
masking (blinding) 34, 61, 65–7, 199–200
matching of subjects 51, 55
McNemar's test 130
mean, arithmetic ($\bar{x}$) 109–10
    self-assessment exercises 116, 120, 227–8, 229
    standard error (SE) 117–19
mean, geometric 113–14
measurement of data
    scales 102–4, 226
    types of data 100–1
median 113, 114
    self-assessment exercises 116, 120, 227, 229
median survival time 176
Medical Subject Headings (MeSH) 10
MEDLINE database 205
membership bias 46
meta-analysis 37, 147–50
    heterogeneity of data 151–4
    publication bias 155–7
meta-regression 154
minimisation (adaptive randomisation) 58–9
missing data 86–90, 176, 200
mode 108, 116, 227
MOOSE group 150
morbidity rates/ratios 83
mortality rates/ratios 82–3, 85, 224
multiple analysis 127, 158

multiple linear regression 52–3, 143
multiple testing 171
multivariate statistics 52–3, 136, 139–44

n-of-1 trials 32
National Guideline Clearinghouse (NGC) (USA) 208
National Institute for Health and Clinical Excellence (NICE) 208
National Library for Health (NLH) 208
negative predictive value (NPV) 167, 169, 172, 230
negligence 192
nested case–control studies 28
Neyman (incidence/prevalence) bias 46
NHS Centre for Reviews and Dissemination (CRD) 208
NHS Economic Evaluations Database (NHS EED) 206
NICE 208
NNH (number needed to harm) 97, 98
NNT (number needed to treat) 94, 97, 98, 99, 174, 225
nocebo response 64
nominal scales 102, 103, 134
nomograms 170
non-inferiority studies 137–8
non-normal distribution 113–15, 132
non-parametric tests 131–2, 141
normal distribution 106–7, 109–12, 133
NPV (negative predictive value) 167, 169, 172, 230
null hypothesis 121–8, 229
number needed to harm (NNH) 97, 98
number needed to treat (NNT) 94, 97, 98, 99, 174, 225

observation bias 45, 47, 48, 65–7, 222
observational analytical studies 25–9, 55, 176–7, 196
    self-assessment exercises 39, 221, 222
observational descriptive studies 24
odds 91, 94, 98, 168, 224, 225
odds ratio (OR) 52, 94, 97–8, 99, 226
off-licence data 217
one-tailed tests 126–7
online resources 12, 150, 205–8, 220

search strategies 9–10, 146
opinion leaders 11, 216–17
opportunity cost 184
OR (odds ratio) 52, 94, 97–8, 99, 226
ordinal scales 102, 103, 134
outcomes (endpoints) 69–77
  see also missing data
Ovid HealthSTAR database 206

P values 122–3, 128, 140, 201
paired t test 133
paired/unpaired data 129, 130, 132, 133
parametric tests 132–3, 141
participant observation 187
Pearson's correlation coefficient (r) 140, 141
peer review 11
PEER value 174
per-protocol analysis 86
percentiles 115
performance bias 45, 46
period prevalence 84
periodicals see journals
Peto method 152
pharmaceutical company representatives 214–17
pharmacoeconomics 180
PICO (analysis of clinical questions) 7–8
pie charts 29
placebos 62–4, 66, 199–200
point prevalence 84
Poisson distribution 106
populations in a study see sample population
positive predictive value (PPV) 166, 169, 172, 230
post-marketing surveillance studies 41
post-test probability/odds 168, 170, 172, 230
power of a study 125–6, 156
PowerPoint presentations 209–11
PPV (positive predictive value) 166, 169, 172, 230
pragmatic trials 22–3
precision (reliability) 70, 74–7, 81
predictive validity 73
presentation skills 209–11
pre-test probability/odds 168, 170, 172, 230

prevalence 84, 85, 224
primary endpoints 69
primary hypothesis 19–20
PRISMA statement 150
probability distributions 105–7
probability (risk) 91–9, 224–5
  in diagnostic tests 168, 170, 172, 230
  significance testing 121–8, 229
prognostic studies 19, 25–6, 175–8
promotional material 216
proportional Cox (hazards) regression 144, 178
prospective studies 25–6, 27
PROSPERO register 150
PsycNET database 206
publication bias 45, 155–7

qualitative data see categorical data
qualitative research 37, 185–9
quality assessment 11–12, 32–5, 146–7, 198–201
quality-adjusted life year (QALY) 182–3
quantitative data 100–1, 102–4, 226
  analytical statistics 129, 131–44
  descriptive statistics 105–7, 109–20, 227–9
  reliability 75
quartiles 114–15
quasi-random allocation 58
quasi-random sampling 43

random sampling 43
random-effects model 152
randomisation 33–4, 51, 56–61, 199
randomised controlled trials (RCTs) 30, 32, 196, 222
  CONSORT checklist 32–5
range 114, 116, 227
ratio scales 103, 134
recall bias 47
receiver operating characteristic (ROC) curves 171–2
reference ranges 107
reflexivity 188
regression 52–3, 141–4, 154
  see also correlation
relative benefit increase (RBI) 96
relative risk (RR) 94, 95–6, 99, 201, 225

relative risk reduction (RRR) 94, 96, 99, 201, 225
  negative 98
reliability (precision) 70, 74–7, 81
reporting bias 45, 155
research pathway for drug development 40–1
resource allocation *see* economic analysis
response bias (observational) 47, 48
response bias (sampling) 46
retrospective cohort studies 26
retrospective studies *see* case–control studies
risk *see* probability
risk factors 25–9
ROC curves 171–2
Rothman's pies 29
RR *see* relative risk
RRR *see* relative risk reduction

safety of drugs 24, 41
sales representatives 214–17
sample population
  allocation methods 33–4, 51, 56–61, 199
  critical appraisal of 199
  matching 51, 55
  restriction criteria 51, 54, 223
  sampling bias 45–6, 48, 222
  sampling methods 43, 187
  size of 125–6, 187
sampling error 46, 119
scale types 102–4, 134, 226
screening studies 164–72, 229–30
SD *see* standard deviation
SE *see* standard error
searching for information 9–10, 146
secondary endpoints 69–70
secondary hypothesis 20
selection bias 45–6, 47, 48, 60, 222
sensitivity (diagnostic tests) 166, 169, 172, 230
sensitivity analysis 88, 154, 184
service provision, audit of 36–7, 212–13, 222
sham treatment 63
SIGLE database (System for Information on Grey Literature in Europe) 206
SIGN (Scottish Intercollegiate Guidelines Network) 196–7, 208
sign test 131
significance testing 121–8, 229
simple randomisation 57
skewed data 113–15
Spearman's rank correlation coefficient (ρ) 141
specificity 166, 169, 172, 230
split-half reliability 76
SQUIRE group guidelines 35
standard deviation (SD) 110–11
  self-assessment exercises 116, 120, 227–8, 229
standard error (SE) 106, 117–19, 120, 156, 229
standard normal distribution 112
standardisation 52
standardised mean difference 112, 126
STARD statement 172
statistical definitions 81
statistical significance 122, 127–8, 201
stratification of data 52
stratified randomisation 57–8
stratified sampling 43
STROBE checklist 28
study design 68
  bias and 44–8, 86, 188, 222
  blinding 65–7, 199–200
  and the clinical question 18–21, 198–9
  clinical trial phases 41
  confounders 49–53, 223
  critical appraisal 33–4, 198–200
  hierarchy of evidence 195–7
  placebos 62–4
  subjects *see* sample population
  types 22–39, 144, 221–2
subgroup analysis 20, 200
subjects *see* sample population
superiority trials 137
surrogate endpoints 69
surveys 37, 185–9
survival analysis 144, 176–8
systematic reviews 37, 145–57
systematic sampling 43

t tests 129, 133
target population 42–3, 199
test–retest reliability 74
thesauri 10

transformation of data 113–14, 115,
    132
treatment studies 19, 30–2, 40–1,
    173–4
TRIAGE website 220
trim and fill method 157
TRIP database (Turning Research Into
    Practice) 206
two-tailed tests 126
type 1 errors (false positives) 20, 90,
    123–4, 124–5, 127
type 2 errors (false negatives) 88,
    124–6, 127

unpaired/paired data 129, 130, 132,
    133
unpublished data 155, 208, 217
Users' Guides to the Medical Literature
    218–19

validity (accuracy) 70, 72–3, 81, 167
variables 81, 134–5
variance (v) 110

washout periods 31
weighted mean 110
Wilcoxon's matched pairs test 132
Wilcoxon's signed rank test 132
worst-case scenario analysis 87

Yates continuity correction 130
Yellow Card scheme 24

z score 111
Z statistic 153
Z test 132

MIDWIFERY PRACTICE GUIDE 7

Core Skills for
Caring and
Assessment

Susan Way

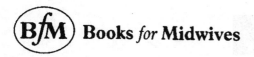

Books *for* Midwives

OXFORD AUCKLAND BOSTON JOHANNESBURG MELBOURNE NEW DELHI

Books for Midwives
An imprint of Butterworth-Heinemann
Linacre House, Jordan Hill, Oxford OX2 8DP
225 Wildwood Avenue, Woburn, MA 01801-2041

℞ A member of the Reed Elsevier plc group

First published 2000
Reprinted 2001

© Susan Way 2000

British Library Cataloguing in Publication Data
A catalogue record for this book is available from the British Library

ISBN 1 898507 73 2

Printed and bound in Great Britain by Athenæum Press Ltd,
Gateshead, Tyne & Wear

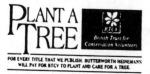

My grateful thanks to:
Patrick, for your patience, understanding, advice and support
Rosie, for those evenings I wasn't home in time to kiss you goodnight
Judy Bradfield, for your artistic talents

CHAPTER 1: **OBSERVATIONS**   page 4

TEMPERATURE
Procedure for taking an oral temperature
Procedure for taking a rectal temperature
Procedure for taking an axillar temperature
Procedure for taking a tympanic temperature

PULSE
Procedure for taking a peripheral pulse

RESPIRATION
Procedure for taking respiration rate

BLOOD PRESSURE
Procedure for measuring blood pressure

CHAPTER 2: **DRUG ADMINISTRATION**   page 29

LEGISLATION

GENERAL PRINCIPLES
Procedure for general drug administration
Administration of a controlled drug
Procedure for administering suppositories
Procedure for administering pessaries
Procedure for the administration of an IM injection
Procedure for the administration of a SC injection
Clinical features which may present in anaphylactic shock

CHAPTER 3: **INFECTION CONTROL**   page 43

CAUSES OF INFECTION

INFECTION CONTROL
When hands need to be washed
Procedure for socially clean hand washing
Four principles of asepsis
Procedure for opening sterile packs
Procedure for putting on sterile gloves

CHAPTER 4: **INTRAVENOUS THERAPY**   page 53

CONTINUOUS INFUSION PUMPS
Calculating the flow rate
Equipment for an intravenous infusion
Procedure for priming the equipment
Connecting the giving-set to the cannula
Changing the infusion container
Technique for removing an intravenous cannula

COMMONLY PRESCRIBED FLUIDS

BLOOD TRANSFUSION
Points to remember when starting a blood transfusion

CHAPTER 5: **VENEPUNCTURE**   page 64

ANATOMY AND PHYSIOLOGY

CARRYING OUT VENEPUNCTURE
Venepuncture procedure

SAFE SHARP PRACTICE

CHAPTER 6: **URINARY INVESTIGATIONS**   page 70

PHYSIOLOGY

OBTAINING A SPECIMEN OF URINE

TESTING A SPECIMEN OF URINE
Points to remember when using reagent strips

URINARY CATHETERISATION
Procedure for urinary catheterisation
Collecting a catheter specimen of urine
Removal of an indwelling catheter

CHAPTER 7: **WOUND CARE**   page 82

PHYSIOLOGY

FACTORS AFFECTING WOUND HEALING

WOUND DRESSINGS
Procedure for changing a dressing
Removal of sutures and clips

WOUND DRAINS
Changing a vacuum bottle
Removal of a wound drain

WOUND ASSESSMENT

CHAPTER 8: **CARE OF THE IMMOBILE WOMAN**   page 93

PRESSURE SORES

THROMBOSIS

RESPIRATORY TRACT INFECTION

PERSONAL HYGIENE CARE
Procedure for a blanket bath

MANUAL HANDLING ISSUES
The shoulder lift

Introduction

This book is intended for use by student midwives and midwives returning to practice after a period of absence. However, midwives in practice would find it useful as a way of refreshing their knowledge about some of the physiology that underpins our practice.

The book covers a number of clinical skills used in midwifery practice that have often been seen as 'nursing skills'. As many midwives today are educated without any nursing background there is a need for books that reflect this approach. *Core Skills for Caring and Assessment* attempts to address this. The skills discussed in this book are those often only referred to in nursing text books and as such are specifically applied to nursing practice. Within this book each chapter links the skills discussed specifically to the childbearing woman and is applied to midwifery practice. Incorporating the physiology provides a basis for understanding the rationale for using certain skills. This in turn, it is hoped, moves away from practices that are viewed at ritualistic.

The procedures identified for performing the skills are written in a step by step approach. This has been done purposefully to give a structure to the student learning the new skill. However, this does not mean it is the only way of doing the skill, and with experience the student will be able to adapt the process to meet the individual needs of the woman and baby.

Many of the skills have similar underlying principles which are pointed out in this introduction, rather than repeating them with every procedure. Firstly, before a procedure is carried out, the appropriate information should always have been discussed with the woman and her partner. This enables an informed decision by the woman when giving consent. The giving of information also includes any procedure that is to be undertaken to her baby. Secondly, dignity and privacy of the woman is paramount during any procedure. Thirdly, any equipment that requires to be disposed of is done so safely with regard to local Trust guidelines. Lastly, all procedures must be documented in the appropriate records, signed and dated. Any abnormalities detected must be refered to the appropriate person.

CHAPTER I

Observations

The measurement of temperature, pulse and blood pressure are often the first clinical procedures which the student midwife is taught. These are all observations which can help with the assessment of the health and wellbeing of a woman and her baby. However, they should not be considered in isolation from the broader clinical picture. For example, a raised temperature (pyrexia) on its own may not be indicative of ill health; the woman may have just drunk a hot cup of tea.

TEMPERATURE

Body temperature represents a balance between heat gain and heat loss. For the body temperature to remain constant, and within the normal range, 36.1°C-37.5°C (Prichard and Mallet, 1992), the relationship between heat loss and heat gain must be maintained.

Temperature constantly alters within a normal range. Generally, it falls to its lowest in the morning and rises to its highest point in the evening. This circadian rhythm, as it is known, produces a maximum body temperature at around 17:00-19:00 hours (Samples et al, 1985). This study concluded that daily observations carried out at this time were sufficient to screen for developing pyrexia, unless other signs and symptoms suggestive of infection were observed at other times.

PHYSIOLOGY

All tissues produce heat as a result of cell metabolism, and this heat is increased by exercise and activity (Marieb, 1989). The internal temperature of the body, the 'core' temperature, is maintained within narrow limits in spite of environmental changes. The actual core temperature is 37°C and does not normally vary by more than 1°C. The core temperature reflects the heat of the arterial blood and represents the heat generated by body tissues in metabolic activity, especially the muscles and liver. Heat loss occurs through the skin via radiation, convection, conduction and evaporation.

The hypothalamus within the brain acts as the body's thermostat, controlling the body's temperature by various physiological mechanisms. It initiates heat-losing activities if the body temperature starts to rise, and heat-gaining activities if the body temperature starts to fall.

If the blood flowing into the hypothalamus is relatively cool, the vasomotor centre becomes excited and there is an increase in sympathetic vasoconstrictor impulses to the skin. The increase in vasoconstriction cuts down heat loss by radiation, conduction and convection. Sweating is also inhibited.

If the temperature of the blood flowing through the hypothalamus starts to rise, impulses are generated which bring about the inhibition of the vasomotor centre. As a result vasodilation occurs due to the arterioles in the skin being stimulated by sympathetic vasoconstrictor impulses. The extra blood passing through the skin warms it, thereby increasing the temperature gradient between the body and it's surroundings, and heat is lost by conduction, radiation and convection. Sweating is also initiated by the hypothalamus.

Hypothermia is a condition in which body temperature drops and the mechanisms used by the body to increase heat production are ineffective. This causes a decline in the metabolic rate and a resulting decrease in all bodily functions. Mild hypothermia is recognised at between 33.1°C and 36°C (Potter and Perry, 1995).

Pyrexia is defined as a significant rise in body temperature. There are various grades of pyrexia:

- Low-grade pyrexia (normal to 38°C) is indicative of an inflammatory response due to mild infection, allergy, disturbance of body tissue by trauma, surgery, malignancy or thrombosis.

- Moderate to high-grade pyrexia (38°C-40°C) may be caused by wound, respiratory or urinary tract infections.

- Hyperpyrexia (40°C and above) may arise because of bacteraemia, damage to the hypothalamus or high environmental temperatures.

A rise in temperature as a result of infection is due to the production of pyrogens. These are released from leucocytes as they become damaged in their work against the invading organisms. The pyrogens reset the body temperature control in the hypothalamus to a higher core temperature. This in turn stimulates a reaction to conserve or manufacture body heat to meet the new set temperature point. Vasoconstriction, inhibition of sweating and shivering occur to raise the body temperature. If at the higher temperature the pyrogens are destroyed, then the thermostat is reset to a lower value and heat-loss mechanisms come into play. Vasodilation occurs, cooling the body back to the level of the reset thermostat. Thus in a fever, periods of shivering and feeling cold are characteristic.

THERMOMETERS AND SITES

The three types of thermometers used for measuring body temperature are mercury-in-glass, electronic and disposable. The mercury-in-glass thermometer is probably the most familiar. The electronic thermometer consists of a rechargeable battery-powered display unit with a temperature-processing probe covered by a plastic sheath. The disposable thermometer consists of a thin strip of plastic with chemically impregnated paper. They are designed for single use, particularly with children, for taking oral or axillary temperatures. The technique and the site used to measure body temperature will depend on the patient, the situation, and the design of the thermometer.

MERCURY-IN-GLASS THERMOMETERS

Core temperature is usually measured at body sites where blood vessels are near to the surface of the skin or mucus membrane. It is essential that thermometer positioning, placement time and environmental factors are all well controlled if an accurate assessment of temperature is to be made.

Oral

This is the most common site used in adults. Its prime advantage is the proximity of the branches of the lingual artery (a branch of the external carotid artery), which makes it an accurate indicator of the core temperature.

Temperatures in the mouth vary considerably. A difference as great as 1.7°C can occur between the cool hard palate and the warm sublingual heat pocket. The heat pockets on either side of the frenulum under the tongue are the areas closest to the sublingual arteries and offer the highest oral temperature.

The mouth should be closed tightly during the monitoring period. Lower readings will be obtained if the mouth is left open, because of air cooling. Tachypnoea (rapid breathing) may also cause a significant reduction in sublingual temperature.

The effects of hot and cold drinks should also be taken into account. Temperatures monitored immediately after drinking iced water have been noted to be significantly lower (Woodman et al, 1967), and the effects can persist for approximately 15 minutes. Hot drinks have a similar effect in altering the temperature and again the effects can last up to 15 minutes. Hot baths have also been found to have an effect (Renbourne, 1963), raising the body temperature by 0.5°C-1.0°C, with a lasting effect of about 45 minutes. Strenuous exercise may also raise core temperature to as high as 40°C.

The length of time a glass thermometer should be left in the mouth has been an area of debate. Whintle (1988) found that the average time student nurses left a thermometer in a patient's mouth was 1.5 minutes, but there was a great deal of variation between first- and third-year students, with the more senior students taking shorter periods of time than first-years. It was noted that students tended to leave the thermometer in the mouth for as long as it took to take the blood pressure and pulse. The more experienced the student was in recording the pulse and blood pressure, the shorter the time for temperature readings.

Closs (1987) examined the recommendations in 27 nursing textbooks and found times considered appropriate for leaving the thermometer in the mouth ranging from 1 to 10 minutes.

A series of studies cited by Closs (1987) showed a mean period of 12 minutes was required to record maximum temperature. However it could be questioned whether a maximum temperature is useful in diagnosing a pyrexia, or whether an optimum temperature is more appropriate. Leaving a thermometer in the mouth for an extra 5 minutes might raise the recorded temperature by 0.1°C, but the significance of the 0.1°C when related to diagnosis and management is probably minimal.

PROCEDURE FOR TAKING AN ORAL TEMPERATURE

- The woman's recent activity is established to ensure that no external factors (as previously identified) could result in a raised temperature.

- The thermometer is checked to ensure the mercury reading is below 35°C.

- The thermometer is placed under the woman's tongue (which she may want to do herself) and she is asked to close her mouth but not to bite on the thermometer.

- The thermometer is removed after the required length of time, and the temperature reading noted.

- The thermometer is cleaned in accordance with local guidelines.

It appears that there is great scope for error, ranging from inappropriate timing to inappropriate positioning of the thermometer. However, if positioning and environmental factors are controlled, then according to Closs (1987), four minutes should give a clinically significant reading.

Rectal

A midwife would probably only use this method with babies. There is increasing resistance to the practice of taking temperatures rectally because of the difficuty in siting the bulb of the thermometer accurately against the rectal mucosa. There is also a risk of perforating the rectum with a poorly positioned thermometer. Some would suggest that rectal temperature taking is contra-indicated in the newborn infant (Potter and Perry, 1995). Also, rectal temperature does not respond as rapidly as a sublingual recording to changes in arterial temperature. The rectal temperature is one degree higher than the oral temperature.

PROCEDURE FOR TAKING A RECTAL TEMPERATURE

- The thermometer is checked to ensure the mercury reading is below 35°C.

- The thermometer must be well lubricated before inserting into the rectum.

- With the non-dominant hand the midwife separates the buttocks to expose the anus.

- The bulb end of the thermometer is gently inserted into the rectum – it must never be forced, and if resistance is met the procedure should be abandoned.

- The thermometer must be held in place by the midwife for approximately 2 minutes (Holtzclaw, 1992) and then removed carefully.

- The thermometer is then wiped and the reading taken, after which the thermometer should be cleansed according to local guidelines.

<u>Axillar</u>

When taking axillary temperatures, the same site, such as the left axillar, should be used on each occasion as variations may be found in the temperature recorded in the right and left axillae. The axillar temperature is one degree lower than the oral temperature.

When using this route for a baby, care is needed to ensure the thermometer stays in place and it is helpful if the baby is quiet and restful.

PROCEDURE FOR TAKING AN AXILLAR TEMPERATURE

- The thermometer is checked to ensure the mercury reading is below 35°C.

- The thermometer is placed into the centre of the axilla, and the arm lowered over the thermometer and placed across the chest. This enables proper positioning of the thermometer against the blood vessels of the axilla.

- It should be left in position for about 3 minutes (Stephen and Sexton, 1987), then removed and read.

TYMPANIC MEMBRANE SENSORS

The tympanic membrane sensor is used exclusively to measure tympanic temperature. An otoscope-like speculum with an infra-red sensor tip detects heat radiated from the tympanic membrane of the ear. As the eardrum is close to the hypothalamus, the recording is sensitive to core temperature changes. This process is quick; within two to five seconds of placement in the auditory canal, a reading appears on the display unit. The ear is an easily accessible site and a rapid measurement can be obtained without disturbing the woman. This is useful when taking the woman's temperature during labour, as the recommended four minutes could well be interrupted by two contractions.

A special neonatal adaptor is required if this method is to be used for the baby.

PROCEDURE FOR TAKING A TYMPANIC TEMPERATURE

■ A clean probe should be used for each woman.

■ The pinna of the ear is pulled straight back and the ear is approached from behind to enable the tip of the thermometer to be directed anteriorly to the tympanic membrane.

■ The probe is placed into the ear, as far as needed to seal the canal.

■ The scanner is turned on and the probe is left in the ear for the length of time that is recommended by the manufacturer.

■ The probe is then removed and the reading recorded.

SKIN THERMOMETER

These are safe to use and non-invasive, but diaphoresis (sweat) can impair the reading. Applied to the forehead or abdomen, the patch changes colour at different temperatures.

APPLICATION TO MIDWIFERY PRACTICE

• To establish a baseline temperature. This is useful as an initial assessment when considering the plan of care for the onset of labour, and as part of the initial examination of the neonate.

• To monitor fluctuations in temperature. This is relevant where a baby has been identified as hypothermic and needs to be nursed in an environment which will increase its body temperature.

• To monitor signs of incompatibility when a woman is having a blood transfusion (see chapter 4).

• To monitor the progress of a woman or baby being treated for an infection.

The measurement of maternal body temperature during the postnatal period is often a routine procedure although it is no longer a statutory requirement. Takahashi (1998) questions its significance in today's practise, arguing that temperature measurement as it stands is not an objective tool for judging a woman's state of health. She suggests that routine checking of maternal temperature in the postnatal period has limited value as a screening test, and a large scale study to evaluate the practice would be valuable.

PULSE

The pulse is a pressure wave of blood caused by the alternating expansion and recoil of elastic arteries during each cardiac cycle (Pritchard and Mallett, 1992). Taking the pulse should be part of an integrated assessment that includes respiration, temperature and, if required, blood pressure.

PHYSIOLOGY

The pulse gives an indirect measurement of heart rate. Each time the heart beats, it propels blood through the arteries, causing the walls of the arteries to expand and distend. The pulse may be felt in any artery that lies near the surface of the body and over a bone or other firm tissue.

The pulse is palpated to assess rate, rhythm and strength (amplitude).

Rate

- An individual with a healthy heart will tend to have a relatively constant pulse rate of around 80bpm.

- Tachycardia is a term used to describe an abnormally fast heart rate, over 100bpm in adults. This may be a result of raised body temperature (perhaps as a result of infection), stress, and certain drugs (such as ritodine hydrochloride).

- Bradycardia is a term used to describe a slow heart rate, under 50bpm (Tortora and Anagnostakos, 1990). This may result from a low body temperature, and certain drugs, but may also be present naturally in fit athletes.

A number of factors can influence a change in the heart rate and therefore the pulse rate. Age is an influencing factor: a newborn baby's heart rate is on average about 140bpm, an infant aged between 1 and 12 months will have a heart rate of approximately 120bpm, and a child aged between 6 and 12 years will have a heart rate of approximately 95bpm.

Pregnancy can also influence the heart rate. In a number of studies, heart rate during pregnancy has been found to increase to between 11% and 17% above pre-pregnant values, peaking at approximately 32 weeks' gestation (McNabb, 1997). This is attributed to a fall in peripheral vascular resistance, which creates a state of relative hypovolaemia. The heart attempts to modify this by an increase in stroke volume (the amount of blood pumped out by a ventricle with each contraction) and hence heart rate.

Heart rate is also affected when the blood volume alters dramatically, for example in the case of a haemorrhage. As the stroke volume declines, cardiac output (the amount of blood pumped out of the ventricle in one minute) can only be maintained if the heart rate is increased.

Rhythm

In a fit and healthy person, the pulse rhythm (the sequence of beats) is regular. That is, the interval between the beats is equal. The pacemaker of the heart (the sinoatrial node) initiates each wave of the heart muscle contraction, and the characteristic rhythm that is results is known as sinus rhythm. Irregular heart rhythms are rarely seen by the midwife, and if detected at a routine assessment the woman should be referred to the appropriate doctor.

Amplitude

This reflects the elasticity of the arteriole wall. A full, throbbing pulse may indicate anaemia (Pritchard and Mallett, 1992) whereas a thin, thready pulse may indicate a loss of circulating blood volume, as with a severe haemorrhage.

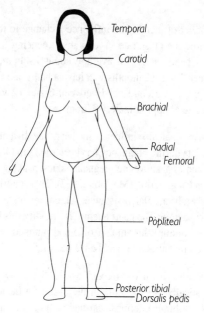

Fig 1.1 **Sites for taking a pulse**

TAKING A PULSE

The pulse may be felt in any artery that lies near the surface of the body and over a bone or other firm tissue (Fig 1.1). It is strongest in the arteries closest to the heart, becomes weaker as it passes through the arterial system and disappears altogether in the capillaries. The radial artery at the wrist is the site most commonly used for determining the pulse, but other arteries that may be used include:

- Common carotid artery, lateral to the larynx

- Brachial artery, along the medial side of the biceps brachii muscle

- Femoral artery, inferior to the inguinal ligament

- Popliteal artery, behind the knee

- Dorsal pedis artery, superior to the instep of the foot.

PROCEDURE FOR TAKING A PERIPHERAL PULSE

- Where possible, measure the pulse under the same conditions each time to ensure consistency.

- The midwife places her second and third finger along the peripheral artery being used to record the pulse and presses gently.

- The pulse should be counted for 60 seconds to detect irregularities or other defects.

Infants under one year of age have small peripheral blood vessels and a rapid pulse rate, which makes counting the radial pulse difficult. The heart rate is variable in the newborn and is influenced by physical activity, crying, state of wakefulness and body temperature (Wieland Ladewig et al, 1994). For accuracy, the heart rate should be assessed both by using a stethoscope and by listening to the apical heart beat (Brunner and Suddarth, 1989). Auscultation is performed over the entire heart region, below the left axilla, and below the scapula. Apical pulse rates are obtained by auscultation for a full minute, preferably when the baby is asleep.

APPLICATION TO MIDWIFERY PRACTICE

- When a baby is born its breathing, colour, heart rate, tone and response to stimuli are all assessed. Any decision regarding resuscitation is based primarily on the first three findings. The heart rate is easily assessed by auscultation or by palpating the chest or umbilical cord (Advanced Life Support in Obstetrics UK, 1996).

- During the postnatal physical examination, the mother's pulse rate is taken for the first few days, and thereafter only if she appears unwell or there are signs of complications such as infection or haemorrhage. A significant rise in pulse rate in either of the above necessitates referral to a doctor (Sweet, 1997).

- Postoperative and critically ill women require careful monitoring of the pulse to assess cardiovascular stability. Hypovolaemic shock following postpartum haemorrhage or caesarean section for example, results in loss of plasma and whole blood, decreasing the circulating blood volume. The resulting acceleration in heart rate causes a tachycardia that can be felt in the pulse rate.

• During the process of labour, a steady pulse rate is an indication that the woman is well. If the rate increases to more than 100bpm it may be indicative of infection or ketosis. It is usual to record the pulse rate every 1 or 2 hours during early labour, and more frequently when labour is more advanced (Cassidy, 1993).

• Women receiving particular drug therapies, such as intravenous ritodine hydrochloride for the management of uncomplicated preterm labour, require pulse monitoring to assess the degree of side-effects that may occur. In the case of a tachycardia over 140bpm the infusion should be ceased (Banister, 1997).

• Women receiving a blood transfusion require careful monitoring of the pulse, as an incompatible blood transfusion may lead to a rise in pulse rate.

RESPIRATION

Respiration is the act of breathing. Its principal purpose is to supply the cells of the body with oxygen and to remove the carbon dioxide produced by cellular activities.

PHYSIOLOGY

For respiration to be effective a number of events must occur:

• ventilation

• gaseous exchange

• internal respiration.

VENTILATION

Breathing in is called inspiration. Just before breathing in, the air pressure inside the lungs is about equal to the pressure of the atmosphere. For air to flow into the lungs, the pressure inside the lungs must become lower than the pressure in the atmosphere. This is achieved by increasing the volume of the lungs. The first step toward increasing the lung size is the contraction of the diaphragm and the external intercostal muscles. Contraction of the diaphragm causes it to flatten, and this increases the vertical dimension of the thoracic cavity. When the external intercostal muscles contract, the ribs are pulled upwards and the sternum is pushed forward. The anterior-posterior diameter of the thoracic cavity is therefore also increased.

Lung tissue is stretched on inspiration which in turn stimulates the afferent fibres of the vagus nerve. These impulses result in inspiration stopping and breathing out (expiration) beginning.

In expiration, the inspiration process is reversed, so that the pressure in the lungs is made greater than that of the atmospheric pressure. Expiration starts when the inspiratory muscles relax, allowing the ribs to move downwards, and the diaphragm returns to its dome shape.

GASEOUS EXCHANGE

Oxygen is carried in the blood in two ways, bound to the haemoglobin within the red blood cells and dissolved in the plasma. Anaemia reduces the oxygen-carrying ability of the blood. As soon as the lungs fill with air, oxygen diffuses from the alveoli into the blood, through the interstitial fluid, and finally into the cells. Carbon dioxide diffuses in the opposite direction, from the cells, through the interstitial fluid to the blood and to the alveoli.

INTERNAL RESPIRATION

This is the exchange of gases that occurs within the tissues between the capillaries and the cells. Carbon dioxide enters the blood and oxygen moves into the cells. Hypoxia is the result of an inadequate amount of oxygen delivered to body tissues.

Respiration is controlled by a number of factors, namely the respiratory centre, nervous control and chemical control. The respiratory centre is located in the brain and is made up of groups of nerve cells. Regular impulses from these nerve cells are sent to motor neurones in the anterior horn of the spinal cord. These neurones supply the diaphragm and the intercostal muscles. When the neurones are stimulated, the muscles contract and inspiration occurs. When the neurones are inhibited, the muscles relax and expiration follows.

If the amount of carbon dioxide in the blood increases, as in the case of exercise, the respiratory centre is stimulated, increasing the depth and rate of respiration. More oxygen is made available to be transported by the blood, and more carbon dioxide is eliminated. Emotion, pain and anxiety can also cause an increase in the respiratory rate (Tortora and Anagnostakos, 1990).

ASSESSING RESPIRATORY RATE

Respiratory observations are carried out to establish a baseline for monitoring change. Respiratory rate does vary considerably in well people, but on average a woman would have a respiratory rate of about 16-20 respirations per minute (rpm). In contrast, the newborn infant would have a respiration rate averaging 40-60rpm. It is important to note any changes in the rate, rhythm or depth from the normal pattern of the woman or baby.

PROCEDURE FOR TAKING RESPIRATION RATE

- If a woman is aware that her respiration rate is being monitored she may become conscious of her breathing and change the rate. To avoid this, the procedure is often done in combination with assessing the pulse rate.

- After palpating the radial pulse the fingers are kept in place and the respiration rate then monitored. One respiration consists of the full cycle of inspiration and expiration.

- The rate is recorded as the number of respirations per minute.

- A baby's respiration rate should not be counted during periods of crying, as this will not reflect the true rate.

In the newborn baby, the breathing is diaphragmatic, with the chest and abdomen rising and falling synchronously. The breathing pattern is erratic with respirations being shallow and irregular, interspersed with brief periods of apnoea (Ho, 1990). The patterns of breathing alter during sleeping and waking.

Respiratory activity can be assessed by observation and inspection. The rate, depth and pattern of the chest-wall movement is observed. General observation of the woman or baby and the effort and sound of breathing provide additional information.

APPLICATION TO MIDWIFERY PRACTICE

Extensive anatomical and functional changes occur in the respiratory system during pregnancy. These changes occur to accommodate the progressive increase in gaseous exchange and the growing space occupied by the uterus.

- Women tend to breathe more deeply during pregnancy. There is a gradual increase in the amount of air inspired and expired with a normal breath. The functional capacity of the lungs increases from 500ml in the non-pregnant state to about 700ml at term.

- There is an increase in oxygen consumption during pregnancy which is facilitated by a 40-50% increase in ventilation and by an 18% increase in the oxygen-carrying capacity of the blood (McNabb, 1997).

- Dyspnoea (undue breathlessness and an awareness of discomfort with breathing) may be a complaint from a woman with severe iron-deficient anaemia (Bewley, 1997).

- Bradypnoea (decreased respiratory rate) can be caused by opiate narcotics, such as pethidine hydrochloride, which depress the respiratory centre (Banister, 1997).

- Respiratory observation is important for critically ill women, during blood transfusion, and on return from theatre.

- Respiratory observation would also be included in the initial and ongoing assessment of the newborn baby.

BLOOD PRESSURE

In the U.K. approximately 80,000 women per annum are diagnosed as hypertensive in pregnancy, before labour starts (Shennan and Halligan, 1996). Consequently, the measurement of blood pressure is an extremely common assessment that the midwife undertakes to assess the health and well-being of the woman during pregnancy. Blood pressure measurements are taken from the very first antenatal visit to the final postnatal discharge check by the midwife.

PHYSIOLOGY

Blood pressure is the pressure exerted by the walls of the blood vessels. The blood pressure depends on cardiac output and peripheral vascular resistance.

Blood Pressure = Cardiac Output x Peripheral Vascular Resistance

Blood pressure is expressed in millimetres of mercury (mmHg) and, unless otherwise specified, blood pressure means systemic arterial blood pressure.

Cardiac output refers to the amount of blood pumped from the left ventricle of the heart per minute. It is calculated by multiplying the stroke volume (the amount of blood pumped out of the heart with each beat) with the heart rate. Cardiac output is measured in litres per minute and is typically around 70ml x 70bpm = 4.9L/min.

Peripheral vascular resistance is resistance exerted by the action of the arteriole walls. The maintenance of a normal blood pressure relies on the balance and adjustment of the systems that modify the factors that produce a cardiac output and the peripheral resistance.

The diameter of the blood vessels is altered with the relaxation or constriction of the smooth muscle wall in the vessel. When the muscle relaxes and the lumen gets larger, this is known as vasodilation. When the smooth muscle constricts and becomes smaller, this is known as vasoconstriction. The action of smooth muscle is influenced by chemical mediators and the nervous system.

Chemoreceptors are sensitive to changes in blood pH or oxygen. When they detect a drop in oxygen tension they send messages to the vasomotor centre which causes vasoconstriction and an increase in blood pressure.

Nerve receptors, known as baroreceptors, sited in the walls of the great arteries such as the aorta and carotid arteries, are stimulated by the stretch of the arterial wall when blood flows through the artery. When the blood pressure rises and stretches the wall, there is an increase in the impulses that the baroreceptors send to the vasomotor centre of the brain. These have an inhibitory effect resulting in vasodilation.

The kidneys also influence blood pressure. The kidney has the ability to increase or decrease the blood volume by controlling the amount of water excreted in the urine. Also, the kidneys release an enzyme called renin, in response to a fall in blood pressure. Renin influences the formation of angiotensin II which is a vaso-constrictor.

Alteration in blood pressure can be due to a number of factors:

- Stroke volume can increase, due to an increase in blood volume, an increase in extracellular fluid retention or obesity. It can also decrease, due to a decrease in blood volume, hypovolaemic shock, septic shock, anaphylactic shock or neurogenic shock.

- Heart rate can be increased by a number of factors including anxiety, pain, excitement, exercise or fever.

- The diameter of the arterioles may increase due to the cold and decrease due to warmth.

- Drugs containing oestrogen, such as the oral contraceptive, may increase the blood pressure, whereas drugs such as lignocaine hydrochloride may reduce the blood pressure.

PROCEDURE FOR MEASURING BLOOD PRESSURE

- Enable the woman to sit comfortably in a quiet environment with her arm resting and supported at heart level. She should rest for at least 5 minutes before the measurement is taken.

- The correct size cuff should be used and restrictive clothing around the arm removed. Placing the cuff over clothing can distort the reading.

- Make sure the centre of the bladder is over the brachial artery and the lower edge of the bladder is above the antecubital fossa.

- Check that the tubing exits from the top of the cuff and so does not interfere with auscultation.

- Place the sphygmomanometer near to you. If a mercury sphygmomanometer is used, the mercury level should be at zero and positioned at eye level, no more than 3 feet away.

- First assess the maximal inflation level by inflating the cuff and palpating the radial pulse at the same time. The level at which the radial pulse disappears is the palpated systolic pulse. Inflate the cuff 30mmHg above this level.

- Locate the brachial artery by palpation and place the stethoscope gently over the point where there is maximal pulsation from the brachial artery. The diaphragm/bell of the stethoscope should not be tucked under the edge of the cuff.

- Release the valve gently, allowing the mercury level to fall slowly and steadily, at about 2mmHg per pulse sound at the normal heart rate.

- Note the systolic pressure at the onset of two consecutive beats (Phase I Korotkoff sounds). Blood pressure should always be recorded in even numbers and read to the nearest 2mmHg on the manometer.

- Record the diastolic blood pressure at KIV or KV, according to hospital protocol.

- If the reading needs to be repeated, wait two minutes before reinflating the cuff to allow the thorough reperfusion of the arm.

CORE SKILLS FOR CARING AND ASSESSMENT

During pregnancy the maternal vascular system undergoes extensive changes which include cardiac output rising by about 40%. This appears to be a response to a fall in systemic vascular resistance. The increase in cardiac output is evident by 8 weeks' gestation, and peaks at about 30 weeks' gestation (de Swiet, 1991). This suggests that systemic vasodilation may be a primary adaptation to pregnancy that initiates a rise in cardiac output, maintaining overall tissue perfusion and blood pressure, prior to significant increases in circulating blood volume (Capeless and Clapp, 1989).

MEASURING BLOOD PRESSURE

Although measuring and monitoring blood pressure is frequently carried out, it is often performed incorrectly, despite being one of the first skills taught to students (Torrance and Serginson, 1996). It has also been noted that teaching is not generally updated nor is knowledge checked (Kemp et al, 1994). The British Hypertension Society's Guidelines on Manual Measurement of Blood Pressure (1993) emphasises the importance of the observer's accuracy as an incorrect reading can lead to the wrong diagnosis. Although it is unlikely that any decision about a woman's care would be made on a single blood pressure reading, there is nevertheless a good argument for sound knowledge and appropriate technique.

Two levels of blood pressure are recorded. The first, the systolic pressure, is the maximum pressure in the vessels during contraction of the ventricles. The second pressure recording is the diastolic, which is the pressure exerted when the ventricles are at rest.

Korotkoff sounds, named after the man who first described them, are sharp, rhythmic knocking sounds that the heart produces with each beat. The sounds become less audible as the flow becomes continuous with the blood in the artery. There are five sounds described in phases:

Phase I   The pressure level at which the first clear tapping sounds are heard

Phase II   The time during inflation when a murmur and a swishing are heard

Phase III   The point where the murmur disappears and a louder and more succinct sound is heard

Phase IV   The point where there is a muffling of sound

Phase V   This is the phase at which the sound disappears

Korotkoff phase V has been argued by many not to be suitable for use during pregnancy because the sound never disappears, so phase IV should be the choice. However, Rubin (1996) argues that there is now sound evidence to support the use of phase V. In a prospective study of 1194 primigravid women blood pressure was measured 5 times at each of 5 different gestation times between 20 weeks and delivery. Among the more than 25,000 readings in the sitting position, phase V was unobtainable in just three. Shennan et al (1996) also found major inaccuracies in the use of phase IV, in that only 16% of recordings were agreed to be the same by both observers recording the blood pressure simultaneously.

The debate continues but if the sound is heard near to zero, then phase IV should be used.

FACTORS WHICH MAY GIVE RISE TO ERRORS WHEN MEASURING BLOOD PRESSURE

With the use of conventional sphygmomanometry, variations due to measurement can occur as a result of instrument error, observer error, or a combination of both.

POORLY MAINTAINED EQUIPMENT

A poorly functioning or incorrectly calibrated manometer can lead to errors of measurement. Sphygmomanometers should be serviced regularly at approximately six-month intervals. The mercury column should be clean, so that the meniscus is clearly visible, and should be calibrated so that the meniscus is initially at zero. The connections should be properly fitting so that air cannot escape. The pump should have a competent working valve that allows a smooth regular release of air.

INACCURATELY PLACED SPHYGMOMANOMETER AND CUFF

The cuff should be placed approximately level with the heart to avoid the hydrostatic effect of a column of blood above or below the heart. The tubing should exit from the top of the cuff so that it does not interfere with auscultation.

CUFF SIZE

Hypertension in obese women may be over diagnosed if the cuff is too small in relation to the woman's arm circumference. The bladder should cover 80% of the upper arm circumference. The recommended bladder dimensions are 13cm x 12.5cm for an adult and 39.5cm x 15.5cm for a large adult. If in doubt, the arm circumference should be measured with a non-distensible tape measure first and the appropriate sized cuff fitted.

RAPID DEFLATION

Rapid or jerky deflation will under estimate and overestimate the systolic and diastolic blood pressure respectively. This may be caused by a poorly functioning control valve. The valve should allow gentle lowering of the mercury at about 2mmHg per second.

MATERNAL POSITION

Errors may occur when different positions are adopted for measuring the blood pressure. In advanced pregnancy especially, lying supine can cause obstruction of the inferior vena cava, resulting in supine hypotension. Blood pressure seems to be lowest when measured in the left lateral position and increases on sitting or becoming upright.

DIFFERENT ARMS

Blood pressure may be different between the left and right arms. It is therefore useful to keep to the same arm for each blood pressure check and to record which arm was used.

CIRCADIAN RHYTHM

Blood pressure can vary considerably throughout the day. There is a circadian rhythm of blood pressure in pregnancy. Highest readings are during the afternoon and early evening, and the lowest during sleep.

TOO COLD

If the woman is cold or the environment is cold, blood pressure rises substantially (*Nursing Times*, 1995). It is important to remember this when considering the measurement, even if there is no way to correct the measurement.

FULL BLADDER

If a woman needs to empty her bladder while waiting for her blood pressure to be measured it can prove another source of error in artificially raising the blood pressure levels (*Nursing Times*, 1995). This is especially of importance for the woman who is having an ultrasound scan as part of her antenatal visit.

DIGIT PREFERENCE

Digit preference and bias are the terms given to the habit of recording blood pressures that end in some specific unit more than others. There is a tendency to record blood pressure to the nearest 5mmHg or 10mmHg, despite the fact that the calibrations on a mercury sphygmomanometer are in 2mmHg.

AUSCULATORY GAP

This is the temporary disappearance of sounds as the cuff deflates. It is quite common with people who have hypertension. This gap can last over 40mmHg and lead to a serious underestimation of systolic pressure and an overestimation of diastolic pressure. This can be excluded by palpating the blood pressure first at the radial artery.

WHITE COAT HYPERTENSION

White coat hypertension has been defined by Shennan and Shennan (1996) as a persistently elevated clinic blood pressure with normal blood pressure at other times. It is found in up to 20% of people with mild hypertension and has been shown to occur in pregnancy (Shennan et al, 1994). It is also known that the presence of a doctor results in higher blood pressure recordings than when a nurse records the measurement (Mancia et al, 1987). It may be useful, therefore, if a midwife with whom the woman is familiar records the blood pressure.

APPLICATION TO MIDWIFERY PRACTICE

- A blood pressure recording is obtained as early in pregnancy as possible in order to determine a baseline measurement. It is then checked at every subsequent antenatal visit.

- Postoperative and critically ill women require monitoring of the blood pressure. Hypovolaemic shock occurring from postpartum haemorrhage or following caesarean section, for example, results in loss of plasma and whole blood, decreasing the circulating blood volume. However, the usual signs of blood loss such as tachycardia and hypotension often appear late in the course of bleeding because of the normal haemodynamic condition of pregnancy, and generally the young age of the woman (Advanced Life Support in Obstetrics Instructors Manual, 1996).

- During the process of labour, the blood pressure is measured every 2-4 hours, then hourly as labour advances (Morrin, 1997). Any changes that may arise in the progress or management of labour (such as the use of syntocinon to accelerate labour, or an epidural for pain relief) may alter the frequency of the blood pressure checks required.

- Women receiving particular drug therapies, such as intravenous ritodine hydrochloride for the management of uncomplicated preterm labour, require blood pressure monitoring to assess the degree of side-effects that may occur.

- Women receiving a blood transfusion require careful monitoring of the blood pressure as an incompatible blood transfusion may lead to hypertension due to the agglutination and haemolysis of red blood cells blocking the kidneys.

References

American Academy of Family Physicians. *Advanced Life Support in Obstetrics Instructors Manual*. University of Wisconsin, 1996.

Banister C. *The Midwife's Pharmacopoeia*. Cheshire: Books for Midwives Press, 1997.

Bewley C. Medical conditions complicating pregnancy. In: Sweet B and Tiran D (Eds). *Mayes' Midwifery: A Textbook for Midwives*. London: Bailliere Tindall, 1997.

British Hypertension Society. *Management Guidelines in Essential Hypertension*. London: British Hypertension Society, 1993.

Brunner L and Suddarth D. *The Textbook of Adult Nursing*. London: Chapman Hall, 1989.

Capeless E and Clapp J. Cardiovascular changes in early pregnancy. *American Journal of Obstetrics and Gynecology*, 1989; 161(6): 1449-52.

Cassidy P. Management of the first stage of labour. In: Bennett, VR and Brown, L (Eds). *Myles Textbook for Midwives*. London: Churchill Livingstone, 1993.

Closs J. Oral temperature measurement. *Nursing Times*, 1987; 83(1): 36-9.

deSwiet M. The cardiovascular system. In: Hytten F and deSwiet M (Eds). *Clinical Physiology in Obstetrics*. London: Blackwell Scientific, 1991.

Ho E. *The Newborn Baby*. Newcastle-upon-Tyne: Atheneum Press Ltd, 1990.

Holtzclaw B. The febrile response in critical care: State of the science. *Heart, Lung* 1992; 21(5): 428-501.

Kemp F, Foster C, McKinlay S. How effective is training for blood pressure measurement? *Professional Nurse*, 1994; 9(8): 521-4.

Mancia G, Parati G, Panidossi G, Rassi G, Casadei R, Zanchetti A. Averting reaction and rise in blood pressure during measurement by physician and nurse. *Hypertension*, 1987; 9: 209-15.

Marieb E. *Human Anatomy and Physiology*. California: The Benjamin/Cummings Publishing Company Inc, 1989.

McNabb M. Maternal and fetal physiological responses to pregnancy. In: Sweet B and Tiran D (Eds). *Mayes' Midwifery: A Textbook for Midwives*. London: Bailliere Tindall, 1997.

Morrin N. Midwifery care in the first stage of labour. In: Sweet B and Tiran D (Eds). *Mayes' Midwifery: A Textbook for Midwives*. London: Bailliere Tindall, 1997.

Nursing Times. Professional development: blood pressure – the role of the nurse, *Nursing Times*, 1995; 91(15): 5-8.

Potter P, Perry A. *Basic Nursing Theory and Practice*. London: Mosby, 1995.

Pritchard A, Mallet J. *The Royal Marsden Hospital Manual of Clinical Nursing Procedures*. 3rd edition. Oxford: Blackwell Scientific Publications, 1992.

Renbourne E. Body heat and clinical thermometry: old concepts and modern ideas. *Current Medicine and Drugs*, 1963; 3(9): 10-31.

Rubin P. Measuring diastolic blood pressure in pregnancy. *British Journal of Medicine*, 1996; 313(7048): 4-5.

Samples J, Van Cott M, Long C, King I, Kersenbrock A. Circadian rhythms: basis for screening for fever. *Nursing Research*, 1985; 34: 377.

Shennan A, Halligan A. Blood pressure measurement in pregnancy: room for improvement. *Maternal and Child Health*, 1996; March: 55-9.

Shennan A, Halligan A, Taylor D, de Swiet M. Defining 'white coat hypertension' using ambulatory blood pressure monitoring. Proceedings from International Society for the Study of Hypertension in Pregnancy, IXth International Congress. *Journal of Hypertension in Pregnancy*, 1994; 13: 339.

Shennan C and Shennan A. Blood pressure in pregnancy: the need for accurate measurement. *British Journal of Midwifery*, 1996; 4(2): 102-8.

Shennan A, Gupta G, Halligan A, Taylor D, de Swiet M. Lack of reducibility in pregnancy of Korotkoff phase IV as measured by mercury sphygmomanometer. *Lancet*, 1996; 347: 139-42.

Stephen S, Sexton P. Neonatal axillary temperatures: Increasing in reading over time. *Neonatal Network*, 1987; June: 25-28.

Sweet B. Postnatal care. In: Sweet B, Tiran D (Eds). *Mayes' Midwifery: A Textbook for Midwives*. London: Bailliere Tindall, 1997.

Takahashi H. Evaluating routine postnatal maternal temperature check. *British Journal of Midwifery*, 1998; 6(3): 139-43.

Torrance C, Serginson E. An observational study of student nurses' measurements of arterial blood pressure by sphygmomanometer and auscultation. *Nurse Education Today*, 1996; 16(4): 282-6.

Torrance C, Serginson E. Student nurses' knowledge in relation to blood pressure by sphygmomanometer and auscultation. *Nurse Education Today*, 1996; 16(8): 397-402.

Tortora G, Anagnostakos N. *Principles of Anatomy and Physiology*. New York: Harper Collins, 1990.

Whintle C. A study of time taken for temperature recordings. Unpublished degree thesis, Bristol Polytechnic, 1988.

Wieland Ladewig P, London M, Olds S. *Maternal-Newborn Nursing*. Wokingham: Addison-Wesley Nursing, 1994.

Woodman E, McConnell P, Simms L. Sources of unreliability in oral temperatures. *Nursing Research*, 1967; 16(3): 276.

CHAPTER 2

Drug administration

Midwives are involved in the administration of medications by a variety of routes and for many different reasons, both in the hospital and in the home. In order to carry out procedures safely and effectively the midwife must have a working knowledge of drug legislation, drug metabolism and procedures relating to drug administration.

LEGISLATION

There are two main items of legislation with which the midwife should be familiar in order to practice safely when administering medicines. These are the 1968 Medicines Act and the 1971 Misuse of Drugs Act.

THE MEDICINES ACT (1968)

The Committee on the Safety of Medicines must have satisfied itself that a preparation is safe and appropriate before it receives a licence. The Act governs all medicinal substances and categorises them as follows:

- *General sales list* (GSL) – these are simple medicines that may be sold by any retailer.

- *Pharmacy only medicines* (P) – these can be sold without prescription but only by a registered pharmacist.

- *Prescription only medicines* (POM) – these can only be obtained when a prescription is issued by a medical practitioner or dentist.

THE MISUSE OF DRUGS ACT (1971)

This governs any drug which is considered addictive or which can lead to misuse. This Act is concerned with the classification of controlled drugs, their possession, supply and manufacture.

THE UKCC (1998:RULE 41)

This states that

A practising midwife shall not on her own responsibility administer any medicine, including analgesics, unless in the course of her training, whether before or after registration as a midwife, she has been thoroughly instructed in its use and is familiar with its dosage and methods of administration or application.

The midwife must also be aware of any contra-indications and side effects, not only to the woman but also to the fetus, or to the baby if the woman is breastfeeding.

Further guidance is given by the UKCC within various booklets it has published (UKCC 1992; UKCC 1998).

DRUG ADMINISTRATION

There are a number of general principles that apply to the administration of any medication.

The administration of a controlled drug within a hospital must involve two persons, one of whom must be a registered midwife. In the majority of cases this would be in preparation for an intra-muscular injection, such as Pethidine. A controlled drug register is

GENERAL PRINCIPLES

- Identify the medicine to be administered on the prescription chart or standing order.

- Check that the medicine has not already been administered.

- Select the appropriate medicine against the prescription chart.

- Check the name of the medicine, the dosage and the expiry date.

- Remove the prescribed dosage from the container.

- Check the prescription and dosage against the medicine container.

- Be certain of the identity of the woman or baby to whom the medicine is to be administered. In hospital this is usually by the identification bracelet hospital number.

ADMINISTRATION OF A CONTROLLED DRUG

- The appropriate drug should be removed from the controlled drug store, and the stock number checked with the number detailed in the register with the second person.

- The date of prescription, the method of administration and the time of administration are noted.

- The stock number of the remaining controlled drugs is also checked and recorded.

- The drug is dispensed and the appropriate details are entered into the controlled drug register.

- Both persons who checked the controlled drug take it to the woman, who is then correctly identified.

- The drug is administered by the appropriate route.

- The controlled drug register is then signed.

kept on each ward or department giving details of stock and administration of controlled drugs. These drugs must be kept in a locked cupboard. The locked cupboard should also be within a locked cupboard, to which the keys are kept by a registered midwife.

After it has been checked that the controlled drug has not already been administered, the following should take place:

The Misuse of Drugs Regulations (1985) provide for the supply of Pethidine to midwives as well its surrender and destruction (UKCC, 1998). In some cases the controlled drug may be supplied to the woman on prescription from a family practitioner. The responsibility for destruction of any unused drugs is that of the mother, to whom in law they belong. The particular drugs, including controlled drugs, which a midwife may use will be determined locally and should be listed in written local policy. Many drugs, however, may be administered by the woman herself, either in the home or if the hospital operates a policy of self-medication.

ORAL PREPARATIONS AND ADMINISTRATION

Giving drugs by mouth is the most frequently used method of administration. Most drugs given by mouth are absorbed into the bloodstream through the walls of the intestines. The speed at which the drug is absorbed and the amount of active drug that is available for use depends upon several factors, including the form in which it is given, for example, whether the drug is in liquid or tablet form, or whether it is taken when the stomach is empty or full.

Some drugs like antacids are taken by mouth to produce a direct effect on the stomach or digestive tract.

Most drugs are specially prepared in a form designed for convenience of administration. This helps to ensure that dosages are accurate and that taking the medication is as easy as possible.

TABLET

This contains the drug compressed into a solid form and is often round in shape. An example of a tablet often taken by a woman, especially in the postnatal period, is paracetamol. This is an analgesic with non-opioid properties and comes under the category of GSL. The usual dose is 500mg-1g, 4-6 hourly up to a maximum dose of 4g daily.

CAPSULE

The drug is contained in a cylindrical gelatin shell that breaks open after the capsule has been swallowed, releasing the drug. A number of different antibiotic preparations come in capsule form. For example, amoxycillin can be administered in capsule form and is maroon/gold in colour. It is a broad spectrum antibiotic often used to treat urinary tract infections, the dosage being 250-500mg tds.

LIQUIDS

The active substance is combined in a solution, suspension or emulsion with other ingredients such as preservatives, flavouring and colouring. Antacids, for example, may be administered in liquid form to reduce gastric acidity and give relief from heartburn. Alginic acid (Gaviscon) is often prescribed for gastric reflux. The dose is usually 10-20mls as required, but the midwife needs to be aware that it impairs the absorption of oral iron.

TOPICAL SKIN PREPARATIONS AND ADMINISTRATION

These are preparations designed for application to the skin and other surface tissues of the body. They include a variety of different types of preparation.

CREAM

A cream can be applied to an area of the body to administer a drug, to cool or to moisten. It is non-greasy and less noticeable than an ointment. Clotrimazole (Canestan) is an antifungal cream and may be prescribed for a woman with candidiasis.

OINTMENT

This a greasy preparation used for applying a drug to the skin or act as a protective lubricant. Anusol ointment is used to relieve the

PROCEDURE FOR ADMINISTERING SUPPOSITORIES

Equipment: Disposable glove
Water soluble lubricant
Drug to be administered

Technique:

- Wash hands and collect together the necessary equipment and drug.

- Ensure that the woman is comfortable in the left lateral position (Sim's position), with her uppermost leg bent towards the waist.

- Unwrap the suppository and apply a small amount of water soluble lubricant at the tip of it.

- Place the tip of the suppository at the rectal entrance and ask the woman to take a deep breath and exhale through the mouth. Gently insert the suppository about an inch beyond the orifice past the internal sphincter.

- It is helpful for the woman to remain on her side for about 15-20 minutes to allow melting and absorption of the medication to take place.

- If the suppository was given to help evacuate the bowel contents then the woman should be reminded where the toilets are located and asked to retain the suppository for as long as possible before she has her bowels open.

effects of haemorrhoids. It should be applied twice daily after a bowel movement, and not to be used for longer than seven days.

RECTAL PREPARATIONS AND ADMINISTRATION

Rectal administration can be for two main reasons, to evacuate the bowel or for drug absorption.

LAXATIVE

These are medicines, also known as aperients, which loosen bowel content and encourage evacuation. They can be given in the form of suppositories or enema. Glycerol suppositories are a GSL preparation and can be prescribed to help relieve constipation. One suppository is equivalent to 4g.

DRUG ABSORPTION

Analgesia can be administered rectally, a route often chosen if a woman is not eating or drinking normally, for instance in the first 12-24 hours following a caesarean section. Diclofenac sodium

---

PROCEDURE FOR ADMINISTERING PESSARIES

Equipment: Disposable gloves
Water soluble lubricant
Drug to be administered

Technique:

- Wash hands and collect together the necessary equipment and drug.

- The woman should be positioned comfortably, usually lying on her back with the shoulders raised (to prevent supine hypotension). The thighs should be separated and the knees bent, but in order to avoid unnecessary exposure the woman can be asked to move and uncover herself when the midwife is ready to begin.

- The midwife washes her hands and puts on a pair of disposable gloves.

- The thumb and finger of the non-dominant hand gently part the labia. The first two fingers of the dominant hand are dipped into some lubricating cream and then gently inserted downwards and backwards into the vagina.

- The pessary is placed into the posterior fornix of the vagina and then the hand removed.

- If, for instance, prostaglandin has been administered then the woman would be required to remain on the bed for about one hour to permit maximum absorption of the drug and facilitate fetal monitoring.

(Voltarol) is a non-opioid analgesic used to help relieve moderate to severe pain. The rectal dose is 100mg, 18 hourly. However, asthma and pregnancy are cited as contra-indications.

VAGINAL PREPARATIONS AND ADMINISTRATION

The drug, when given vaginally, is absorbed via the vaginal mucosa. Dinoprostone (Prostin E2), is one such preparation which is used in the induction of labour to ripen the cervix. The usual dose is 1-2mg depending on parity, and Bishop's Score. This can be repeated 6 hourly, but staff are often guided by the hospital protocol for dose and frequency of administration.

INJECTION PREPARATION AND ADMINISTRATION

An injection is the act of giving medication by use of syringe and needle (Pritchard and Mallet, 1992). The three most common types of injections used in obstetrics are:

- Intravenous (IV)
- Intramuscular (IM)
- Subcutaneous (SC).

Several factors will determine the choice of route of administration.

INTRAVENOUS ROUTE

Speed of action is greatest with an intravenous injection. The drug is delivered into a systemic vein and within seconds will be returned to the heart. It will then be rapidly delivered to all parts of the body. Although the effect is rapid, so also are any side-effects or adverse reactions.

The IV route is essentially painless, especially if a cannula is already in situ. This is particularly advantageous if regular doses are to be given.

It is generally agreed that the IV drugs can only be administered by the midwife after she has undertaken further training in this particular area following qualification. Therefore, for the purpose of the rest of this chapter only IM and SC injections will be considered.

INTRAMUSCULAR ROUTE

In the adult the intramuscular route is usually selected because the muscle can accept larger volumes than subcutaneous tissue; up to 5mls of fluid may be introduced into one site. Irritant drugs are less likely to cause abscesses or necrosis and absorption is more rapid and reliable than via the oral or subcutaneous route. The skeletal muscles are well perfused with blood and have relatively few pain receptors.

The most common types of drugs that are injected via this route are analgesics, antiemetics and antibiotics. When considering the newborn baby, the most common drug likely to be administered via this route is Konakion.

SUBCUTANEOUS ROUTE

The speed of action is slower, and the duration of the effect longer, when compared to the intramuscular route. This is because the blood supply to the adipose layer is relatively poor, so systemic absorption is correspondingly delayed. The most common drugs the midwife will be involved in administering via this route are insulin, heparin and possibly some vaccines.

INTRAMUSCULAR INJECTIONS

In the adult there are three main sites that may be used with intramuscular injections (Fig 2.1).

VASTUS LATERALIS MUSCLE

This area is the anterior lateral aspect of thigh. The thigh is divided into three equal lengths and the injection given into the middle segment on the outer aspect. The right or the left side of the body may be used. This is a useful site as it is free from major nerves or blood vessels. It is also a large muscle and can accommodate repeated injections.

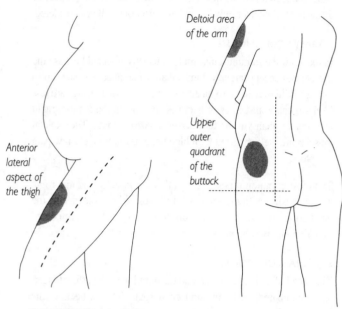

Figure 2.1 **Site for injection**

GLUTEUS MUSCLE

This area is the upper outer quadrant of the buttock and can tolerate injections of large volumes. However it is not an ideal injection site as there is the risk of sciatic nerve damage and low absorption rate. The gluteal muscles are very underdeveloped in the baby and should not be used as an injection site until the child has been walking for about a year (Wong, 1995).

DELTOID MUSCLE

This area is only suitable for small volumes of fluid (<2ml) but has a rapid absorption rate. Because the area is small it limits the number of injections that can be given at this point.

For an IM injection to be successful an important factor is the choice of needle. The needle must be long enough to traverse the skin and subcutaneous tissue and deposit the drug well into the muscle. If the needle is too short the injection will go into subcutaneous fat. Absorption will be disrupted and irritant drugs will cause more trauma in fat.

It is important the appropriate size syringe for the amount of drug to be administered is used as well as the correct size needle. For example, the choice of syringe and needle will be very different if administering Pethidine to a woman in labour, when compared to giving a newborn infant Konakion.

PROCEDURE FOR THE ADMINISTRATION OF AN IM INJECTION

Equipment: Clean receiver
Needle
Syringe
Drug to be administered
Prescription sheet/standing order

Technique:

– The chosen site for the injection is exposed.

– The non-dominant hand stretches the skin around the site to facilitate the insertion of the needle and to displace the subcutaneous tissue.

– With the dominant hand, the needle is held at an angle of 90° and quickly plunged into the skin. This will ensure the muscle has been penetrated.

– Approximately a third of the shaft of the needle is left exposed which will facilitate removal of the needle if it breaks.

– The plunger is pulled back slightly. If no blood is aspirated the plunger is depressed slowly. This will help prevent pain and ensure even distribution of the drug. If blood appears when the plunger is initially drawn back, then withdraw the needle completely, replace it and begin again.

– Following the complete administration of the drug, the needle is withdrawn rapidly and pressure is applied to any bleeding point. This will help prevent haematoma formation.

The routine technique of cleansing the skin before administering an injection, by rubbing the area briefly with an alcohol impregnated swab, has been identified as being of little value (see Chapter 5).

SUBCUTANEOUS INJECTIONS

The common sites used for this procedure are the upper outer aspect of the arm, the outer aspect of the thigh and the abdomen. Theoretically, however, almost any site is possible. Rotation of these sites decreases the likelihood of irritation and ensures improved absorption.

PROCEDURE FOR THE ADMINISTRATION OF A SC INJECTION

Equipment: Clean receiver
Needle
Syringe
Drug to be administered
Prescription sheet/standing order

Technique:

- The chosen site for the injection is exposed.

- With the non-dominant hand the skin is grasped firmly to elevate the subcutaneous tissue.

- With the dominant hand the needle is inserted into the skin at an angle of 90° and then the grasp is released.

- The plunger is pulled back slightly. If no blood is aspirated the plunger is depressed slowly. This will help prevent pain and ensure even distribution of the drug. If blood appears when the plunger is initially drawn back, then withdraw the needle completely, replace it and begin again.

- Following the complete administration of the drug, the needle is withdrawn rapidly and pressure applied to any bleeding point. This will help prevent haematoma formation.

Tachycardia and possible arrhythmias
Anxiety and agitation
Sneezing
Husky voice
Facial oedema
Flushing and redness
Itchy urticarial wheals
Gastrointestinal symptoms
Shock (acute hypotension), often causing collapse
Bronchospasm leading to brochoconstriction
Upper airway oedema with possible laryngeal spasm

POTENTIAL COMPLICATIONS
WHEN ADMINISTERING DRUGS

- Local and systemic allergic or hypersensitivity reactions may occur. All known allergies should be recorded appropriately in the woman's maternity notes and if in hospital, on her drug chart. Before giving a drug, the woman should be asked about known allergies or previous adverse reactions. Anaphylactic reactions usually occur within a minute or two of the drug being given, but may be delayed for up to half an hour.

- There is a possibility of administering the drug into inappropriate tissue, the biggest danger being of an IM preparation being given IV. This is why the plunger of the syringe must always be withdrawn before being depressed to inject the drug, to ensure a blood vessel has not been punctured.

- Nerve damage is possible with poor technique but should not occur if the site is selected correctly.

- Pain is probably an inevitable consequence when having an injection administered. With careful attention to technique, the pain of IM injections can be greatly reduced. The pain will either be cutaneous, due to the receptors in the skin, or muscular. Muscle is not normally sensitive to the needle, but contains pressure receptors which can respond when the drug is injected.

ANAPHYLACTIC SHOCK

This is an acute hypersensitive drug reaction. It usually occurs suddenly, in less than an hour after the drug has been administered, but within minutes if it has been given IV (Laurence and Bennett,, 1992). Treatment is urgent and death may occur.

Any hospital ward or other place where anaphylaxis may be expected should have all the drugs and tools necessary to deal with it in one convenient pack. Each student should quickly become familiar with the local protocols and policies which cover such an emergency and seek adequate training in resuscitation techniques.

References

Beyer Blodget, J. Managing injection reactions. *Nursing 95*, 1995; 25(9): 46-7.

Laurence D, Bennett P. *Clinical Pharmacology*. London: Churchill Livingstone, 1992.

Pritchard A, Mallet J. *The Royal Marsden Hospital Manual of Clinical Nursing Procedures*. 3rd edition. Oxford: Blackwell Scientific Publications, 1992.

UKCC. *Standards for the Administration of Medicines*. London: UKCC, 1992.

UKCC. *Midwives Rules and Code of Practice*. London: 1998.

Wong D. *Whaley and Wong's Nursing Care of Infants and Children*. 5th edition. St Louis: Mosby, 1995.

Further reading

Banister C. *The Midwife's Pharmacopeia*. Cheshire: Books for Midwives Press, 1997.

Briggs G, Freeman R, Yaffe S. *Drugs in Pregnancy and Lactation*. 3rd edition. London: Williams and Wilkins, 1990.

CHAPTER 3

Infection control

Most of the women midwives come into contact with are fit and healthy women. However, on occasions they will encounter women who are vulnerable to the risk of developing an infection. The immune system of the baby is immature so is at risk of developing an infection from invading organisms.

With these factors in mind it is important for the midwife to understand the main causes of infection and how to prevent or minimise its spread. The midwife should also be familiar with local guidelines, policies and procedures for infection control.

CAUSES OF INFECTION

An infection can be defined as the deposition and multiplication of bacteria and other organisms in tissues or on surfaces of the body where they can cause adverse effects (Ayliffe et al, 1992).

Simply by coming into hospital, women risk being exposed to Hospital Acquired Infections (HAIs). This risk can be further exacerbated if a woman has in any way lost the integrity of her skin, for example as a result of an intravenous infusion, an episiotomy or a perineal tear.

Hospital Acquired Infection is also known as a nosocomial infection. It can be defined as an infection found in a patient in hospital that was not present and was not being incubated on admission, or an infection which, having been acquired in hospital, appeared after the patient was discharged (Ayliffe et al, 1992). It is a major problem in all hospitals, with massive financial implications.

There are many reasons why infections spread so easily in hospital, but the main ones include laxity in hand washing between clients, and the careless handling of soiled articles. Hospitals should have infection control policies in place to prevent the transmission of infection. Infection control however, may have become a ritualised routine of little value. Walsh and Ford (1989) argue that much nursing practice in this area is ritualistic and back up their arguments with convincing detail. There is nothing to suggest that midwifery practice is any different.

PHYSIOLOGY

The development of an infection depends on three key factors:

- The number of organisms entering the body.
- The virulence of the invading organism.
- The resistance of the host.

In certain conditions, organisms are able to multiply rapidly. They may be able to survive over a wide range of temperatures, and do not always need oxygen. An organism requiring oxygen to survive is known as aerobic; organisms which do not require oxygen are anaerobic. Organisms do not generally survive well in dry areas, in places where nourishment is lacking, or in places which are very acidic or alkaline.

The more virulent the organism, the more serious the disease. Virulence depends upon the biological characteristics of the organism, its mode of action and the toxins (if any) that are produced. As virulent organisms multiply rapidly, they may also produce mutations, which also have an effect on virulence. Non-pathogenic organisms may become pathogenic (potentially disease-producing) through mutation. It is known that certain bacteria which have undergone mutation have developed resistance to various antibiotics, such as penicillin and tetracycline.

The resistance of the host to organisms varies widely among individuals. Factors such as stress which may accompany surgery, bereavement, or an important event, tend to lower resistance. Nutritional status, adequacy of blood supply and age may also cause a reduction in the body defence system. Preterm and newborn babies are at risk because many of their natural defences are not fully developed.

TRANSMISSION OF INFECTION

- Transmission can occur by direct contact, where the organism is passed on directly by contaminated equipment or by the hands of the midwife.

- Organisms can be carried through the air in dust or on skin scales; for example this may occur during bed making if sheets are shaken.

- Blood borne transmission, where blood or blood stained material transmits the organism, can happen with needle-stick injuries, existing breaks in the skin, sexual activity or potentially from mother to baby.

- Food poisoning occurs when contaminated food is ingested.

Individuals are protected from organisms by the body surface and by internal mechanisms. The body surface includes the skin, mucus membranes and certain bodily secretions such as sebum from the sebaceous glands. Internal protective mechanisms include the inflammatory response and the production of antibodies.

The woman or baby may become infected via a number of routes. These include via a breakage in the skin, for example from perineal trauma, or a fetal scalp electrode site; via the alimentary tract if hygiene is poor when making up a bottle feed; via the genito-urinary tract, perhaps because of repeated catheterisations; and via the respiratory tract.

ORGANISMS OF PARTICULAR CONCERN

METHICILLIN-RESISTANT STAPHYLOCOCCUS AUREUS (MRSA)

Staphylococcus aureus is part of the normal human flora, with large numbers of organisms existing on the skin and mucosa. However, if the organism enters the body it can cause a serious systemic infection, such as a major wound infection, pneumonia or septicaemia. MRSA is able to spread easily from person to person, often on the hands of staff. Some strains of MRSA have the ability to spread hospital wide, and it has proven impossible to eliminate them from hospitals.

HUMAN IMMUNODEFICIENCY VIRUS (HIV)

The myths and misconceptions surrounding HIV are rampant within the health care professions. Gallagher (1990) identified that even after an education programme, irrational fears were still held about contracting AIDS (Acquired Immunodeficiency Syndrome).

Within midwifery, an area of high risk from blood contact, transmission of HIV from an individual to a health care worker during a clinical procedure is very rare. In order to maintain confidentiality, avoid discrimination and ensure safe working practices, all staff should adopt Universal Infection Control Precautions when handling blood and all blood-stained body fluids, irrespective of the serological status of the individual and regardless of any suppositions made about them (Kennedy and Edwards, 1993). Gloves should be worn whenever handling a placenta, and when handling a baby until it has been bathed to remove amniotic fluid and blood. Women should be taught and encouraged to take responsibility for the careful and hygienic disposal of their own soiled materials.

INFECTION CONTROL

The principles of controlling the spread of infection fall into three categories (Office of Health Economics, 1997, Ayliffe et al, 1992).

1 Remove the sources or potential sources of infection, which

includes treatment of infected individuals as well as sterilising, disinfecting and cleaning contaminated materials and surfaces.

2 Block the transfer of bacteria from those potential sources to infected individuals. This includes such measures as hand washing, aseptic operations, and 'non-touch' dressing techniques.

3 Enhance the individual's resistance to infection, for example by using prophylactic antibiotics for a woman who is having an emergency caesarean section (Enkin et al, 1995).

HAND WASHING

Blowing the nose, visiting the toilet and handling soiled nappies are some of the actions that result in significant hand contamination. Hand washing is a simple yet effective way to help prevent the spread of infection.

Good hand washing technique, covering all surfaces of the hands at the right time, is more important than what the hands are washed with or the length of time the hands are washed. Sadly, it seems to be a forgotten technique. A recent report from the Public Health Laboratory on Hospital Acquired Infection (Glynn et al, 1997) showed that hand washing before or following some procedures

---

AS IDENTIFIED BY GOULD (1997) AND HORTON (1995), HANDS NEED TO BE WASHED BEFORE:

- Performing invasive procedures.

- Preparing or handling food.

- Before and after any aseptic procedure.

- After handling items that may be or are soiled.

- Coming on and off duty.

- After going to the toilet, blowing or touching one's nose.

was lacking and that written policy regarding hand washing may not be followed in practice. Larson and Killien (1982) refer to a number of reasons for non-compliance including:

- The health professional is too busy.
- The health professional does not believe that they are at risk of acquiring infections from patients.
- The hand washing agent is detrimental to the skin.
- The health professional is wearing gloves.
- The sink is inconveniently located.

PROCEDURE FOR SOCIALLY CLEAN HAND WASHING

- The hands are moistened and then soap or skin disinfectant rubbed into them.

- The palms are rubbed together vigorously in order to remove dead cells and bacteria.

- The entire surface of both hands should receive contact, including the interdigital spaces.

- Wrists, thumbs and fingernails need to be cleaned.

- All surfaces should be rinsed thoroughly and then dried with a paper towel. The friction caused by the paper towel helps remove any remaining bacteria.

- The whole process should take about 15-30 seconds.

Social hand washing, that is washing the hands for 10-15 seconds with plain soap and running water and mechanical friction (this being the most important element of hand washing), is intended to render the hands socially clean and is sufficient for many midwifery activities both on healthcare premises and in the woman's home.

Taylor (1978) identified areas of the hand that were most likely to be forgotten in the hand washing procedure. These included parts of the thumb, finger tips and palms of the hand.

Mild detergents and emollients are the most commonly used hand cleaners, enabling organisms to be easily removed by washing for 10-15 seconds. Alcohol-based cleansers have an important role, especially when access to facilities is difficult or inconvenient, for example when it is necessary to perform a procedure urgently in the neonatal unit and there is no time to wash the hands properly. Antiseptic cleansers include chlorhexidine and povidone iodine preparations. It is believed (McLure and Gordan, 1992) that povidone iodine preparations have a wider spectrum of activity than chlorhexidine, even against MRSA. Antiseptic skin cleansers are useful where it is known that the patient is vulnerable to infection from resident organisms.

Clear, concise guidelines on hand washing have been developed by the Infection Control Nurses' Association in association with the medical skin care hygiene company Deb (Rees, 1997). It is hoped that the national guidelines will provide a framework on which to build improved hand washing with clear, concise, educational information on all aspects of hygiene.

Some general points to consider are:

• Finger nails should be kept short; avoid wearing rings and watches (Gould, 1997).

• Cuts should be covered with occlusive waterproof dressings to reduce the risk of blood borne infections such as hepatitis B and HIV.

• Cloth towels, often favoured in doctors' surgeries and in the home, can promote cross-infection especially if damp and not laundered daily.

• Hot air dryers circulate air loaded with bacteria.

It is recommended that disposable gloves are worn when in contact with bodily fluids (Royal College of Nursing, 1992), but gloves are not an alternative to hand washing. Hands should be washed following removal of gloves. The RCN (1992) also recommend that aprons are worn to protect clothing when contamination or splashing of clothing with water or bodily fluids may occur. This is especially important for those midwives who no longer wear a prescribed 'hospital uniform'.

ASEPSIS

Sterility means the absence of micro-organisms. Sterilisation can be accomplished by a number of different methods such as boiling, use of various chemicals and autoclaving (steam under pressure). Some things cannot be sterilised, notably human skin. However, items that cannot be sterilised must be cleaned thoroughly and disinfected as much as possible.

THERE ARE FOUR BASIC PRINCIPLES OF ASEPSIS:

- Know what is sterile.
- Know what is not sterile.
- Store sterile equipment correctly.
- Remedy contamination immediately.

Even when using sterile items, the midwife must be aware of what is not sterile. Contamination occurs when a sterile surface comes in contact with any unsterile surface. This can occur by accidentally touching the sterile surface with hands or an unsterile object.

Most health settings use pre-packaged sterile kits, packs and supplies. When using these sterile supplies, the outer layer or wrapping must be inspected to ensure it is intact, without visible holes, tears or damage. Paper and plastic materials used for wrapping must be impervious to dust and resistant to moisture.

When the outer wrapping of a sterile surface touches a non sterile surface, it is no longer sterile. It is also considered (Rambo, 1985) that once the outer wrapping is opened, the outer inch edge of any sterile field is also contaminated because airborne micro-organisms may have settled on it.

PROCEDURE FOR OPENING STERILE PACKS

■ The pack is taken to the area where it is to be used. This may involve the use of a cleaned trolley if in the hospital or a table top if in the home. The outer wrap is then removed

■ The hands are washed as previously described.

■ The sterile pack is opened, being careful to avoid contamination.

■ Remember always face the sterile field, or go around the sterile field if necessary.

■ Allow sufficient space (at least 12 inches) between your body and the sterile field.

■ Individually wrapped supplies, such as needles and syringes should be opened according to the manufacturer's instructions. This is often by grasping the package by the slightly extended edges provided and peeling along the sealed edge.

■ The article is then handed to the 'sterile' person keeping fingers away from the edges.

PROCEDURE FOR PUTTING ON STERILE GLOVES

■ Wash the hands.

■ Open the pack so the sterile gloves are visible.

■ Pick up one glove, touching only the edge of the cuff.

■ Pull on the glove.

■ Pick up the second glove with the gloved fingers under the cuff.

■ Pull the second glove on with other hand.

■ Continue pulling the gloved cuff up over the wrist.

■ Pull the other glove up over the wrist.

■ Adjust the fingers of the glove as necessary.

When wearing sterile gloves, hands should be kept in sight, away from unsterile objects and above waist level. The sterile area is generally considered to be confined to the trolley or table top and above waist level. Anything that hangs, falls or touches below these levels is considered contaminated.

The floor is recognised as a contaminated area. Clean or sterile items that fall on the floor should be discarded or decontaminated. Any portion of a sterile drape or equipment that hangs below a table top is considered unsterile. The outside of glass vials and ampoules containing medication is also unsterile. Contamination can occur when reaching across or above a sterile field with bare hands or arms or with non sterile items. Coughing or sneezing over a sterile field will result in it becoming contaminated and so must be avoided.

As a midwife, when transporting sterile equipment in the car in preparation for a home birth, for example, it is important that the packaging does not become damp or damaged in any way. The storage of sterile equipment is important; it should be kept on a clean dry surface.

References

Ayliffe G, Lowbury E, Geddes A, Williams J. *Control of Hospital Infection: A Practical Handbook*. 3rd edition. London: Chapman & Hall, 1992.

Enkin M, Keirse M, Renfrew M, Neilson J. *A Guide to Effective Care in Pregnancy & Childbirth*. 2nd edition, Oxford: Oxford University Press, 1995.

Gallagher R. AIDS: the fear of contagion. *Nursing Times*, 1990; 4(19): 30-2.

Gould D (1997). Practical procedures for nurses No.1: Handwashing. *Nursing Times*. 1997; 93(37).

Glynn A, Ward V, Wilson J. *Hospital Acquired Infection Surveillance: Policies and Practice*. London: Public Health Laboratory Service, 1997.

Horton R. Hand washing: the fundamental infection control principle. *British Journal of Nursing*, 1995; 4(16): 926-32.

Kennedy J, Edwards S. HIV infection in the midwifery setting. *Modern Midwife*, 1993; 3(3): 25-9.

Larson E, Killien M. Factors influencing hand washing behaviour of patient care personnel. *American Journal of Infection Control*, 1982; 10: 93-9.

McLure A, Gordan J. In vitro evaluation of povidone-iodine and chlorhexidine methicillin-resistant Staphylococcus aureus. *Journal of Hospital Infection*, 1992; 21: 291-9.

Office of Health Economics. *Hospital Acquired Infection*. London: OHE, 1997.

Rambo B. *Nursing Skills for Clinical Practice*. Volume 3. London: W B Saunders, 1985.

Rees J. Washing instructions. *Nursing Times*, 1997; 93(37).

Royal College of Nursing. *Guidelines on Infection Control for Nurses in General Practice*. London: RCN, 1992.

Taylor L. An evaluation of hand washing techniques (part 1). *Nursing Times*, 1978; 74(2): 54-5.

Walsh M, Ford P. *Nursing Rituals: Research and Rational Action*. Oxford: Heinemann, 1989.

CHAPTER 4

Intravenous therapy

An intravenous infusion (IVI) is the introduction of prescribed sterile fluid into the blood circulation (Jamieson et al, 1997).

A woman being attended by a midwife may require an IVI for a number of reasons:

- To maintain a normal fluid, nutrient and electrolyte balance when she is unable to maintain this adequately by herself, for example, following a caesarean section.

- To maintain a normal fluid, nutrient and electrolyte balance when it has been recommended to restrict the fluid and diet intake of the woman, for example, when labour is classed as high risk.

- To replace sudden and excessive blood loss in an emergency situation. If a woman is having a severe postpartum haemorrhage with hypovolaemic shock, rapid replacement of fluid is necessary.

- To administer medication when other routes are inappropriate. Syntocinon infusion when augmenting or accelerating labour is such an example.

- To pre-load the circulatory system to reduce the risk of hypotension, prior to the siting of an epidural.

The above indications would generally be classed as short-term, that is, the infusion would only be expected to last for a few hours or a couple of days at most. In this instance therefore, it is usually the veins of the back of the hand or the superficial veins of the wrist or lower arm that are chosen as the infusion site.

The decision to commence an IVI is usually that of the medical practitioner, who would prescribe the therapy on the appropriate intravenous prescription chart. There may be local Trust differences so it is important that midwives refer to the policies and guidelines relevant to their own practice.

A midwife may encounter an emergency situation, especially in the community setting, where the decision to site an IVI would be hers. Therefore, a midwife who has the clinical expertise to site an IV infusion may save valuable time and possibly lives.

Most prescribed fluids are commercially prepared in sterile containers and they are labelled for intravenous infusion. They may also be prepared by the hospital pharmacy. The containers used for these preparations are frequently soft plastic bags protected by an outer covering.

Administration sets are commercially prepared in sterile packs. The set contains specialised sterile tubing; at one end there is a rigid trocar protected by a sterile sheath. At the other end is a similarly protected Luer connector nozzle. Towards the trocar end, the trocar widens into a drip chamber. An adjustable roller clamp surrounds the tubing below the drip chamber, which allows the flow of fluid to be regulated at the prescribed flow rate. Blood administration sets include a filter.

Various cannulae are available, and are prepared commercially in sterile packs. They usually have an inner needle surrounded by a plastic cannula. The needle is withdrawn once the vein is punctured, allowing blood to flow back. Once the cannula is safely in situ the infusion fluid is connected and the cannula is secured in position. Small winged needles are used for access to veins in babies.

CONTINUOUS INFUSION PUMPS

Continuous infusion pumps are common and are generally the preferred method for controlling the precise amount of fluid to be infused, over a specific period of time. There are a variety of products on the market which can be broadly categorised according to their mode of action (Woollons, 1997).

GRAVITY DRIVEN PUMPS

These operate using gravity as the method of infusion and deliver fluid at a very low pressure. The drip rate is counted by an electronic sensor and they are only suitable for the administration of low-risk infusions (in which overload of the drug is not a critical factor).

ELECTRONIC PUMPS

Fluid delivered is under positive pressure and this can be a safe and reliable means of delivery. Volumetric pumps deliver a pre-determined volume of fluid over a specific period of time. Due to their complex technology they can be used to deliver high risk infusions where overload is a risk factor. Peristaltic pumps describe the action of the infusion sets. They usually incorporate the same features as the volumetric pumps.

Syringe pumps usually range from 5-60 ml and are suitable for the administration of high-risk infusions needing to be delivered at a slow rate, for example, maintaining the dose for a continuous epidural infusion.

MECHANICAL PUMPS

These are particularly useful for ambulatory use, are lightweight and do not require an external power source.

CALCULATING THE FLOW RATE

If an infusion pump is not being used then the number of drops per minute required needs to be calculated accurately in order to maintain the flow of infusion at the prescribed rate.

All administration sets include details of the number of drops per ml for that particular set, known as the drop factor. Using this information the flow rate can be calculated accurately.

$$\frac{\text{Total volume of infusion} \times \text{Drop factor (see administration set)}}{\text{Total time of infusion in minutes}}$$

Example

Total volume of fluid = 500ml

Time for completion = 4 hours, i.e. 240 mins (4 × 60 mins)

Drop factor = 15

$$\frac{500\text{ml} \times 15 \text{ (drop factor)}}{240 \text{ minutes}} = 31.2$$

= 30 drops per minute (approx.)

Thus the number of drops required to maintain the infusion at the required rate = 30 per minute when the drop factor is 15.

EQUIPMENT FOR AN INTRAVENOUS INFUSION

- Clinically clean trolley or tray
- Sterile dressing pack, if required
- Appropriate size cannula – to cause the minimum discomfort but permit the optimum flow rate (usually grey colour, size 16FG allowing 170 ml/min to flow)
- Alcohol-based antiseptic for cleansing the skin
- Gloves
- Sterile administration set
- Prescribed sterile infusion fluid
- Sterile transparent dressing
- Infusion stand
- Tourniquet
- Hypoallergenic tape
- Receptacle for soiled disposables
- Local anaesthetic and equipment for its administration
- Continuous infusion pump

The position of the cannula in the vein and the movement of the woman's limb may have an effect on the flow rate. It is important to assess visually the rate of fall of fluid in the infusion container as well as to regulate the required drops per minute. For example, when the time for completion is four hours, one quarter of the fluid should have been infused after 1 hour, and half the fluid after two hours. Other factors which may affect the flow rate include the tubing of the administration set becoming pinched or kinked, and occlusion of the cannula due to formation of a clot.

Priming the equipment for intravenous infusion involves preparing the prescribed infusion fluid by running it through the administration set. Appropriate hand washing and asepsis should be maintained during this part of the practice to prevent contamination.

The equipment should not be primed until immediately before the infusion to minimise the risk of infection. When siting the cannula, the non-dominant limb of the woman should be used if possible. This will hope to minimise her discomfort by allowing freedom of movement of her dominant hand. It is important to read the manufacturer's instructions for priming the infusion set, as there may be slight variations with the technique.

Once the cannula has been sited and taped into position, the midwife needs to be ready to connect the primed administration set to the cannula.

Once the infusion is connected and the correct rate is being infused, continuing care will include observing the cannula site to ensure the cannula remains securely fixed. The site should also be inspected regularly for signs of phlebitis (inflammation of the vein), leakage and infection.

Within a 72 hour time span the empty containers can be replaced with full containers of prescribed infusion fluid without changing the administration set. The evidence available suggests that the optimal time interval for the replacement of IV giving-sets is every 72 hours.

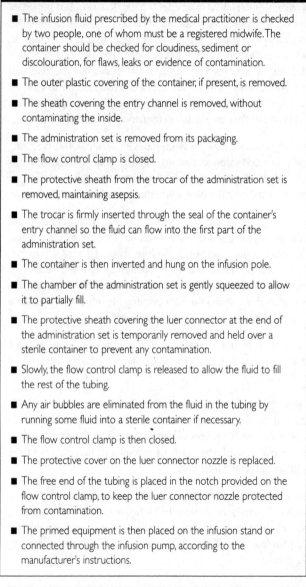

PROCEDURE FOR PRIMING THE EQUIPMENT

- The infusion fluid prescribed by the medical practitioner is checked by two people, one of whom must be a registered midwife. The container should be checked for cloudiness, sediment or discolouration, for flaws, leaks or evidence of contamination.

- The outer plastic covering of the container, if present, is removed.

- The sheath covering the entry channel is removed, without contaminating the inside.

- The administration set is removed from its packaging.

- The flow control clamp is closed.

- The protective sheath from the trocar of the administration set is removed, maintaining asepsis.

- The trocar is firmly inserted through the seal of the container's entry channel so the fluid can flow into the first part of the administration set.

- The container is then inverted and hung on the infusion pole.

- The chamber of the administration set is gently squeezed to allow it to partially fill.

- The protective sheath covering the luer connector at the end of the administration set is temporarily removed and held over a sterile container to prevent any contamination.

- Slowly, the flow control clamp is released to allow the fluid to fill the rest of the tubing.

- Any air bubbles are eliminated from the fluid in the tubing by running some fluid into a sterile container if necessary.

- The flow control clamp is then closed.

- The protective cover on the luer connector nozzle is replaced.

- The free end of the tubing is placed in the notch provided on the flow control clamp, to keep the luer connector nozzle protected from contamination.

- The primed equipment is then placed on the infusion stand or connected through the infusion pump, according to the manufacturer's instructions.

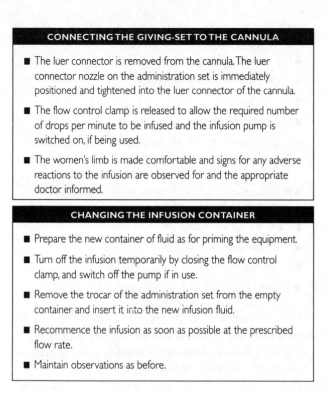

CONNECTING THE GIVING-SET TO THE CANNULA

- The luer connector is removed from the cannula. The luer connector nozzle on the administration set is immediately positioned and tightened into the luer connector of the cannula.

- The flow control clamp is released to allow the required number of drops per minute to be infused and the infusion pump is switched on, if being used.

- The women's limb is made comfortable and signs for any adverse reactions to the infusion are observed for and the appropriate doctor informed.

CHANGING THE INFUSION CONTAINER

- Prepare the new container of fluid as for priming the equipment.

- Turn off the infusion temporarily by closing the flow control clamp, and switch off the pump if in use.

- Remove the trocar of the administration set from the empty container and insert it into the new infusion fluid.

- Recommence the infusion as soon as possible at the prescribed flow rate.

- Maintain observations as before.

Preparation for changing a container should begin when the midwife notices that there is only a small amount of fluid remaining in the infusion container. This allows the container to be exchanged before the level of fluid drops below the point of the trocar in the neck of the container, thus preventing the formation of air bubbles in the system and the dangers of air embolus. Removal of the intravenous cannula is performed using an aseptic technique.

COMMONLY PRESCRIBED FLUIDS

HARTMANN'S SOLUTION

Hartmann's solution has a similar composition to that of human plasma but contains no bicarbonate ions and has a significant concentration of lactate. The lactate enables the support of extra

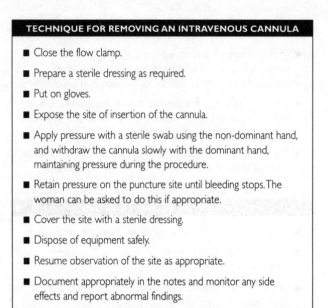

TECHNIQUE FOR REMOVING AN INTRAVENOUS CANNULA

- Close the flow clamp.
- Prepare a sterile dressing as required.
- Put on gloves.
- Expose the site of insertion of the cannula.
- Apply pressure with a sterile swab using the non-dominant hand, and withdraw the cannula slowly with the dominant hand, maintaining pressure during the procedure.
- Retain pressure on the puncture site until bleeding stops. The woman can be asked to do this if appropriate.
- Cover the site with a sterile dressing.
- Dispose of equipment safely.
- Resume observation of the site as appropriate.
- Document appropriately in the notes and monitor any side effects and report abnormal findings.

cellular bicarbonate concentration but with the reduced risk of circulatory overload. Hartmann's solution is often the preferred choice of fluid when an epidural is sited.

NORMAL SALINE

Normal saline (sodium chloride 0.9%) is widely used to sustain extra cellular fluid volume, compensating for losses due to such factors as haemorrhage during surgery. Sodium chloride is found predominantly within extracellular fluid so any saline infused will increase the volume of these fluids. Normal saline is often used when the intravenous therapy is short term.

RED CELLS, WHOLE BLOOD (BLOOD TRANSFUSION)

Each unit contains 450mls of whole blood. The two main reasons for giving a blood transfusion are an acute haemorrhage where sudden hypovolaemia needs to be corrected, or if the haemoglobin level falls below a certain value. The latter is often a cause for debate as many fit, healthy women are able to tolerate a large degree of haemodilution before being symptomatic. The temperature storage for whole blood is between 2°C to 6°C and it has a shelf life of 35 days.

BLOOD TRANSFUSION

Dangerous or fatal transfusion errors are usually caused by failure to keep to standard procedures (McClelland, 1996). It is therefore essential to follow local guidelines and procedures.

Acute haemolytic transfusion reactions are usually caused by transfusing red cells that are incompatible with the individual's ABO blood type. They usually result from errors made in identifying the individual when samples are being taken or when blood is being transfused (McClelland, 1996).

A number of blood tests may be undertaken in anticipation of requesting blood for a transfusion, such as prior to an elective caesarean section or when caring for a woman at high risk of having a severe postpartum haemorrhage.

GROUP AND SAVE

When a group and save is requested on the blood form, the sample of the woman's blood that is sent to the laboratory will have its ABO and Rh D type determined. Also, the serum is screened for IgG antibodies that could damage red cells at 37°C. Following this, the serum sample is then held in the laboratory for a short period of time, usually about seven days. If the red cells are required within this time, a further test to exclude ABO can be rapidly performed, and within approximately 15 minutes blood is ready to issue to the woman.

CROSSMATCH

When this request is made, the transfusion department tests the blood sample for compatibility with the red cells from the units of blood that are to be transfused. Compatible units of blood are then labelled specifically for the woman and kept for 48 hours for immediate use.

BLOOD TRANSFUSION: POINTS TO REMEMBER

■ Each hospital will have its local guidelines and procedures which should be followed.

■ The compatibility report which is provided by the hospital transfusion centre (often with the first unit of blood to be transfused) should be identified and checked. The woman's full name, ABO and Rh D group as well as a unique donation number is on the report.

■ The compatibility report should be checked against each unit of blood when it is ready to be transfused, for the name of the woman, date of birth and hospital number, ABO and Rh D group, unique donation number and the date and time for which the blood is requested.

■ The information on the woman's hospital identity bracelet is checked against the compatibility label and report.

■ The expiry date of the blood pack is checked as well as for leakages or damage to the pack.

■ A base line set of observations including temperature, pulse and blood pressure should be taken and recorded, for future reference.

■ During the transfusion the temperature, pulse and blood pressure should be taken and recorded according to local policy. Any adverse signs and symptoms such as vomiting, itching, headache and severe loin pain should also be observed for, all being potential signs of blood incompatibility. The infusion must be stopped if they occur and a medical practitioner informed.

■ A fluid balance chart is required and needs to be maintained.

■ The flow rate on the giving set should be adjusted to achieve the infusion rate over the prescribed period of time.

■ No other infusion solutions or drugs should added to any blood products and all blood needs to be transfused through a blood transfusion giving set containing an integral filter.

■ The longest time whole blood should take to be infused is 5 hours as it should not be away from the controlled temperature environment for longer than this period of time.

References

Jamieson E, McCall J, Blythe R, Whyte L. *Clinical Nursing Practices*. 3rd edition. London: Churchill Livingstone, 1997.

McClelland D (ed). *Handbook of Transfusion Medicine*. 2nd edition. London: HMSO, 1996.

Woollons S. Selection of intravenous infusion pumps. *Professional Nurse Supplement*. 1997; 12(8): S14-5.

CHAPTER 5

Venepuncture

Venepuncture is the term used for the procedure of entering a vein with a needle.

Venepuncture is carried out for 2 main reasons:

- To obtain a blood sample for diagnostic purposes.
- To monitor levels of blood components.

Within midwifery practice, venepuncture is primarily used to collect blood samples for diagnostic purposes. This could be at any time during the antenatal, intrapartum or postnatal period. In early pregnancy, for example, blood is taken to determine the haemoglobin level, Rhesus status, blood group and presence of Rubella antibodies, to provide a basis for planning the appropriate care and management with the woman. During intrapartum care the midwife may be required to take a blood sample from a woman known to be Rhesus negative, to estimate the number of fetal cells in the maternal circulation. During the postnatal period the midwife may be required to assess the haemoglobin level of a woman demonstrating signs and symptoms of anaemia.

ANATOMY AND PHYSIOLOGY

The commonest site for venepuncture is the antecubital fossa because it has a selection of superficial veins strongly supported by the surrounding musculature (Inwood, 1996). The usual choice is the basilic vein, the cephalic vein or the median cubital vein (Fig 5.1). Veins in the dorsal aspect of the hand may be used if difficulty is encountered with the veins in the anticubital fossa.

Fine veins, and veins that are thrombosed from previous procedures, should be avoided. An area that is bruised or adjacent to a site of infection should also be avoided. If the woman complains of pain or soreness over a particular site, this should not be used either.

Use of veins which cross joints or bony prominences and those with little skin or subcutaneous cover, e.g. the inner aspect of the wrist, will subject the woman to more discomfort.

Palpation should be the primary method of vein selection, although it is more straightforward if the vein can also be seen. The area should be palpated from side to side to assess for suitable veins. Palpation is also of value in distinguishing structures clinically, for example arteries and tendons, due to the presence of a pulse or the feeling of resistance and for detecting deeper veins.

The left arm is normally used in a right-handed woman. However, if a suitable vein is not found in one arm, the other arm needs to be assessed.

The tunica media, the middle layer of the vein wall, is composed of muscle fibres which are capable of constricting or dilating in response to stimuli from the vasomotor centre in the medulla via the sympathetic nervous system. There are a number of factors which may influence this response of which the midwife needs to be aware.

ANXIETY
This may be reduced by a calm confident manner and by explanation of the procedure. Careful preparation and an unhurried approach should aid relaxation for the woman.

TEMPERATURE
If the woman is cold, the veins may not be evident on first

inspection. The application of heat may be useful, either by applying a warm compress or by soaking the arm in warm water.

CARRYING OUT VENEPUNCTURE

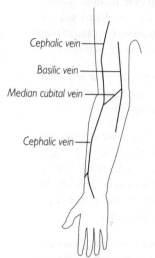

Cephalic vein

Basilic vein

Median cubital vein

Cephalic vein

Fig 5.1 **Selection of vein**

As a general rule, in adults a 21-gauge (green) needle should be used. This enables blood to be withdrawn at a reasonable speed without undue discomfort to the woman. Slower drawing of the blood would give it more time to clot in the needle. A smaller bore needle may cause increased haemolysis of the blood due to damaging the blood cells.

There are several vacuum systems available that leave the needle in place while the different specimen containers are attached. The containers are pre-vacuumed to draw up the volume of blood required for the test.

POTENTIAL RISKS TO THE WOMAN

• The needle may inadvertently be pushed through a valve in the vein which usually causes greater pain than would ordinarily be caused by venepuncture.

• Inadequate cleansing of the skin may allow bacteria to enter the skin and cause phlebitis, which may be painful and can damage the vein.

• If the midwife 'overshoots' the vein a haematoma usually forms.

• The brachial artery may be inadvertently punctured, resulting in the blood flow coming out in a pulsating motion and appearing bright red in colour. To stem the flow from an artery, direct pressure needs to be applied for anything up to 5 minutes.

VENEPUNCTURE PROCEDURE

Equipment: Clean receiver

Appropriate size needle and syringe or vacuum set

Correct blood bottles

Blood request forms

Alcohol impregnated swab or other method of cleansing the skin if appropriate

Dressing

Non-sterile gloves

Procedure:

- Where appropriate it may be necessary to offer counselling to the woman about more specific blood tests such as HIV and fetal screening.

- The arm should to be fully supported to ensure comfort.

- Adequate lighting is necessary to enable the arm to be seen properly.

- Apply the tourniquet at a pressure that is greater than venous and lower than arterial blood pressure. This allows blood into the arm but stops it leaving, causing the vein to fill with blood.

- Encourage the woman to open and close her fist, maintaining the arm in an extended position. This encourages the veins to become prominent. The vein may be tapped gently, promoting blood flow and therefore vein distension.

- Select a vein which should feel hard and bouncy.

- Put on gloves.

- The skin can be cleaned using an alcohol impregnated swab. If this method is used the skin should be given time to dry before the needle is inserted. This will facilitate coagulation of the organisms, thus enhancing disinfection (Pritchard and Mallett, 1992).

- Anchor the vein by applying traction on the skin a few centimetres below the proposed insertion site. This immobilises the vein facilitating smooth entry of the needle.

- The needle should be inserted along the line of the vein at an angle of 15° for about 1-2cm before the blood is withdrawn.

▶

> - Allow the vacutainer bottles to fill as required or withdraw the appropriate volume of blood via the syringe. Take care when removing and changing bottles to prevent dislodging the needle.
> - Loosen the tourniquet to decrease the pressure in the vein. This will help prevent bleeding and bruising when the needle is removed.
> - Place a sterile swab over the entry site but do not press.
> - Remove the needle carefully.
> - When the needle has been removed apply pressure at the entry site for 2 minutes to stop the bleeding. This can be done by the woman herself. The arm should not be bent as this will cause a shearing force to be applied to the hole in the vein, enlarging it and causing more bleeding and bruising.
> - If blood is to be transferred from a syringe into blood specimen bottles it should be done without forcing it out of the syringe as this may cause haemolysis and give rise to inaccurate results.
> - Ensure the specimen bottles have been labelled correctly. Citrate bottles may be rolled to ensure mixing.
> - Inspect the puncture site before applying a sterile adhesive dressing if necessary.

SAFE SHARP PRACTICE

Needle-stick injuries pose a hazard to health care workers. Goldwater et al (1989) reported one needle-stick injury for every 3175 to 4006 needle-handling procedures. Needles should not be resheathed and must be disposed of in the appropriate sharps receptacle. This applies equally to procedures undertaken by the midwife in the woman's home. Whoever uses the sharps should be responsible for disposal of the equipment.

In the event of injury the wound should be encouraged to bleed by, for example, squeezing the edge of the puncture site to milk out as much blood as possible, or by holding the wound under running water (Royal College of Nursing, 1990). The Occupational Health Department should be informed and details of the incident completed in accordance with local policy.

References

Goldwater P, Law R, Nixon A. Impact of recapping device on venepuncture-related needle-stick injury. *Infection Control and Hospital Epidemiology*, 1989; 10(1): 21-5.

Inwood S. Designing a nurse training programme for venepuncture. *Nursing Standard*, 1996; 10(21): 40-2.

Pritchard A, Mallett J. *The Royal Marsden Hospital Manual of Clinical Nursing Procedures*. 3rd edition. Oxford: Blackwell Scientific Publications, 1992.

Royal College of Nursing. *Acceptable Sharp Practice*. Video. London: Healthcare, 1990.

Further reading

Campbell J. Making sense of the technique of venepuncture. *Nursing Times*, 1995; 91(31): 29-31.

Rowland R. Venepuncture. *Nursing Times*, 1991; 87(32): 41-3.

CHAPTER 6

Urinary investigations

The examination of urine can be a valuable aid to diagnosis and screening for several conditions in pregnancy and childbirth. The midwife may therefore be involved in testing a specimen of urine in the home, clinic setting or ward environment. It should always be seen as part of the holistic care offered to the woman, rather than as a routine task divorced from client care.

PHYSIOLOGY

The main function of the urinary system is to help keep the body in homeostasis by controlling the composition and the volume of the blood. Toxic wastes and excess essential materials are removed from the body, primarily in the form of urine. The major part of this process is carried out by the nephrons.

Urine formation requires three principal processes:

- glomerular filtration
- tubular reabsorption
- tubular secretion.

Glomerular filtration involves the forcing of fluids and dissolved substances through a membrane at high pressure. When blood enters the glomerulus, the blood pressure forces water and dissolved substances through the endothelial pores of the capillaries, basement membrane and through into the Bowman's capsule. The pressure required to filter the blood may be affected by certain conditions. These include kidney disease, where the glomerular capillaries increase their permeability, letting plasma proteins through, and severe haemorrhage which produces a drop in the general blood pressure. A dramatic drop in blood pressure may result in no filtration occurring.

As the filtrate passes through the renal tubules, about 99 percent of it is reabsorbed into the blood. Only about 1 percent of the filtrate actually leaves the body. This is known as tubular reabsorption. The process is very discriminating and only specific amounts of substances are reabsorbed, depending on the body's needs. Substances that are reabsorbed include water, glucose, amino acids and ions such as sodium, potassium and calcium.

When the sodium concentration of the blood is low, there is a drop in blood pressure, and the renin-angiotensin pathway becomes activated. In response to the low blood pressure the juxtaglomerular cells of the kidneys secrete an enzyme called renin which converts angiotensinogen into angiotensin I. When angiotensin I passes through the lungs, it is converted into angiotensin II. Angiotensin II, an active hormone, causes constriction of the efferent arterioles of the kidneys resulting in an increase in glomerular blood pressure. This ensures normal filtration pressure at the glomerulus. The presence of angiotensin II also results in aldosterone being secreted by the adrenal cortex, bringing about an increase in sodium and water reabsorption by the distal convoluted tubules.

Tubular secretion adds substances to the filtrate from the blood. This process enables the body to be rid of certain materials as well as helping to control the blood pH. The body has to maintain normal blood pH (7.35-7.45). The normal diet often provides more acid-producing foods than alkali-producing foods (Tortora and Anagnostakos, 1990). To raise blood pH, the renal tubules secrete hydrogen ions into the filtrate, which makes the urine acidic.

Prior to the collection of a specimen of urine the woman should be informed of the following:

- Why the test is being carried out.

- How to collect the sample.

- What container is to be used if one is not supplied by the midwife.

- If not in the home, where the toilet and washing facilities are located.

- Who to give the specimen of urine to, if it is not the midwife.

- When the specimen is required.

- Instruct the woman to collect the specimen directly into a sterile universal container, once the flow of urine has been established and before the bladder is empty.

- Transfer the specimen into the appropriate sterile specimen collecting container (as per hospital policy) and send it to the laboratory appropriately labelled, with an accurately completed request form, within the hour.

The results of the urine test should be recorded accurately in the woman's records, as soon as possible after testing. A negative result on a particular date may be significant in retrospect, so all results should be recorded.

TESTING A SPECIMEN OF URINE

When testing a specimen of urine the same precautions for infection control should be practised as for handling any bodily fluids. These include wearing a disposable apron if clothing is likely to be soiled, and using disposable gloves if body fluids are to be touched (RCN, 1992).

If the specimen is not tested within an hour of collection it should be kept refrigerated, and should be allowed to warm to room temperature before being tested (Cook, 1996). This is because bacteria in the urine may multiply, causing changes in the pH and altering the composition of other constituents of the sample, which may confuse results. For these reasons, the midwife should ask the woman to bring a fresh specimen of urine to the clinic or to provide a specimen on arrival.

Prior to testing a specimen of urine, there are a number of observations that should first be made:

APPEARANCE

The urine should be straw coloured. Colour changes, such as red colouring, may be due to contamination with blood, which could occur following a 'show' at the onset of labour, or perhaps lochial loss during the postpartum period.

ODOUR

Normal, freshly voided urine has very little smell. If left to stand, it develops an ammoniacal smell. A sweet smell is due to the excretion of acetone, which occurs with ketoacidosis. This may be from a woman, for example, whose diabetes mellitus has become poorly controlled in pregnancy, or from an anorexic woman who has been starving herself. Infected urine may have a characteristic fishy smell on voiding which becomes worse when left to stand.

TESTING URINE USING A REAGENT STRIP

A number of substances may be detected on routine testing of urine with a reagent strip. The reagent strip should be dipped briefly into a fresh, well-mixed specimen of urine, so that all the reagent areas are immersed, and then removed immediately. A clock, or a watch with a second hand should be used to time when the strip is removed from the specimen, as for accurate results, the reading of the reagent blocks must be done at the specified time intervals. The colours of the reagent blocks are compared with the colour chart on the bottle label, remembering to keep the strip horizontal to ensure no mixing of colours between the reagent blocks. After testing, the urine should be discarded in a sluice or toilet, and the reagent strip disposed of in a clinical waste bag.

POINTS TO REMEMBER WHEN USING REAGENT STRIPS

- The reagent strips must be stored as per manufacturer's instructions.

- The reagent strips should be stored in the bottle supplied.

- The bottle cap should be replaced as quickly as possible after removing a reagent strip for use.

- The bottle should be stored in a cool, dry place but not refrigerated.

- Reagent strips should not be used after the expiry date.

PH VALUE

The pH of urine indicates how acid or alkaline it is. A value of 7.0 indicates a neutral solution, below 7.0 is acidic and above 7.0 is alkaline. A normal pH value for urine is 5.0-6.0 but can vary from 4.8-8.5 (Bayer Diagnostics, 1996). Values are usually lowest after an overnight fast and highest after meals. A reading below this level could indicate that a woman's metabolism has become too acidic due, for example, to ketoacidosis resulting from poor diabetic control. A pH above 7.0 is most likely to be a urinary tract infection.

PROTEIN

Protein in urine can indicate a urinary tract infection, or perhaps, when a rise in blood pressure has been noted, signify pregnancy induced hypertension with proteinuria. A trace of protein may be found with rupture of the membranes (Cassidy, 1993). Transient positive results are not always significant, as the receptacle may have been contaminated, or the specimen may have contained leucorrhoea.

GLUCOSE

This is not normally found in the urine of a non pregnant woman. During pregnancy, however, it can be a common feature and may signify a change in renal function rather than carbohydrate metabolism (Boyle, 1994), demonstrating the normal lowered renal threshold of pregnancy. If glycosuria persists, serum screening for diabetes mellitus should be carried out.

KETONES

Ketones are the by-products of the breakdown of fatty acids and usually occur in either starvation or diabetes mellitus. If ketones are present in the urine during pregnancy a woman may be suffering from morning sickness, may have an erratic dietary intake, or may be trying to lose weight. Diabetes mellitus should be considered as a possible cause.

BLOOD

Blood should not be in urine. If blood is found to be present in the urine the midwife needs to determine if the specimen was contaminated. With discussion it may be revealed that the woman has been bleeding rectally due to haemorrhoids, or it could be that she is suffering from the symptoms of a urinary tract infection. In the early postnatal period it may be difficult to collect a clean specimen of urine due to the presence of lochia.

NITRITES

These are not normally present in urine and are produced when gram negative bacteria, such as E. coli, convert dietary nitrates to nitrites. E. coli is responsible for 80% of urinary tract infections (Enkin et al, 1996), and the presence of nitrites is strongly suggestive of an infection.

URINARY CATHETERISATION

A catheter is a hollow tube that can be used to remove fluids from, or instil fluids into, a body cavity or viscus. Urethral catheters are designed for insertion into the urinary bladder.

Common indicators for short-term catheterisation (less than 14 days) in midwifery practice include:

- Drainage of urine postoperatively, for example following a caesarean section.

- Accurate measuring of urine output during acute illness. This may be necessary if a woman had severe pre-eclampsia or had suffered a very large blood loss.

- Retention of urine. A woman may be unable to void urine during labour if she has an epidural in situ.

- Risk of trauma to a full bladder during an operative procedure. Prior to commencing a caesarean section an indwelling catheter would be inserted to ensure the bladder remains empty during the operation.

There are two types of catheterisation:

- Intermittent.
- Indwelling.

INTERMITTENT CATHETERISATION

Catheters used for this procedure are generally made from latex or plastic. The procedure involves the insertion of a single channel catheter into the bladder, which is then removed when the bladder has been emptied of urine. Within midwifery practice this is usually performed prior to an instrumental delivery, to avoid trauma to the bladder, or for the relief of urinary retention, for example during labour, when the woman is unable to void urine spontaneously.

INDWELLING CATHETERISATION

The Foley catheter is probably the best known. It is a self-retaining, flexible latex tube. It has two interior channels, one for drainage and one for balloon inflation. It is retained in the bladder by means of the balloon which is inflated after insertion.

PROCEDURE FOR URINARY CATHETERISATION

Equipment: Catheter and bag
Syringe and needle
Sterile water
Sterile catheter pack
Sterile gloves
Cleansing solution
Catheter stand

Technique:

- Ensure there is a good light source available to enable the vulval area to be seen clearly.

- Assist the woman into the supine position, ensuring she is tilted laterally if pregnant, usually on her left side to an angle of about 15°. This will reduce the risk of supine hypotension. The knees should be bent, with hips flexed and feet resting approximately 60 cm apart.

- If appropriate ask the woman to remove the sanitary towel, observing any 'show', liquor amnii or lochia.

- An aseptic technique is used throughout (see chapter 3). Wash hands and put on sterile gloves.

- Position the water repellent towel underneath the woman's buttocks.

- Using a downward movement, swab each side of the labia majora, then the labia minora using antiseptic lotion. Use each swab only once and then discard.

- Introduce the tip of the catheter into the urethral orifice in an upward and backward direction and advance the catheter until 5-6cm have been inserted. If difficulty is encountered while introducing the catheter, the sterile gloved forefinger of the other hand should be inserted into the vagina and placed along the anterior wall. The tip of the catheter can then be felt and if it is directed parallel with the finger in the vagina, the catheter will enter the bladder without injury to the urethra (Cassidy, 1993). If the catheter is obstructed by the fetal head, upward pressure on the head by the finger in the vagina will allow passage of the catheter.

▶

▶

> - Allow the bladder to empty, collecting the urine in the sterile container.
> - Remove the catheter when urinary flow ceases or inflate the balloon according to the manufacturer's directions.
> - Connect the catheter to the drainage system.
> - Secure the drainage catheter or drainage system to the thigh. Care must be taken not to occlude the lumen of the catheter or to cause excessive constriction of the limb. Traction of the catheter should also not occur.
> - Make the woman comfortable.
> - Collect a urine specimen for examination if required and measure the amount of urine collected.

The choice of drainage equipment depends upon the reason for catheterisation. For a woman who is recovering postoperatively from a caesarean section, a single one or two litre bag with or without an outlet tap, supported on a stand or by a hanger on the bed frame would be appropriate. However, a woman requiring a high degree of dependency care with severe pre-eclampsia, would require a drainage bag incorporating a urine measure device, so hourly recordings of urine output could be made.

CATHETER AND BALLOON SIZE

The catheter size is measured in Charriere (Ch) or French gauge (Fg) units. These are equivalent to 0.33mm and refer to the external diameter of the catheter: 12Ch = 4mm external diameter. The optimal gauge for a woman is 12-14Ch (Gould, 1994). Fitting a larger gauge catheter than required may cause irritation to the urethral mucosa leading to leakage and pain.

Most indwelling catheters are now provided with a 5-10ml balloon capacity. Larger balloon size is associated with increased bladder irritability (Kennedy et al, 1983).

COLLECTING A CATHETER SPECIMEN OF URINE (CSU)

This is the collection of a specimen of urine for microbiological analyses, from a woman who has an indwelling catheter in situ.

Equipment: Catheter clamp
Gloves
Cleansing solution
Needle and syringe
Specimen container
Laboratory request form

Technique:

- The drainage bag tubing is clamped below the sample port and left for approximately 15 minutes to allow urine to accumulate. Urine samples should not be taken from the drainage bag as it may contain a higher concentration of micro-organisms.

- Wash the hands and put on gloves.

- Cleanse sample port with an alcohol saturated swab, allow to dry.

- Insert the assembled needle and syringe at a 45° angle to the sample port and withdraw the urine sample.

- Remove the needle and syringe and empty the collected specimen of urine into the appropriate sterile container.

- Remove the clamp to allow the urine flow to be re-established.

- Place the specimen container into the specimen bag and attach the appropriate laboratory request form.

- Ensure the labeled specimen is transported to the laboratory immediately.

COMPLICATIONS OF CATHETERISATION

TISSUE DAMAGE AND INFLAMMATION

This can be minimised with the use of appropriate techniques for insertion and removal of the catheter as well as the correct choice of material and size, latex and PVC being the most appropriate for short-term use. Further risk of damage may be avoided by providing effective support for the drainage bag, and by emptying the bag before it becomes too heavy and drags on the catheter.

INFECTION

Catheterisation can increase the risk of urinary tract infection (UTI) in three different ways. Organisms can be picked up by the catheter during insertion and carried to the bladder. Organisms may migrate along the peri-urethral space between the external surface of the catheter and the urethral surface. Finally, organisms may travel up the lumen of the catheter following entry, either at the junction between the catheter and the bag collecting tube, or into the bag via the drainage tube.

There are a number of precautions that can be taken to reduce the incidence of infection. Any handling of the catheter bag can be a potential source of cross-infection. Hands should therefore be washed and dried thoroughly before and after any procedures. Gloves should be worn, to avoid any contact with body fluids.

REMOVAL OF AN INDWELLING CATHETER

Equipment: Non-sterile gloves
Measuring jug
Syringe

Technique:

– The woman should be instructed to use the bidet prior to removal of the catheter.

– Collect a CSU if required.

– Assist the woman into the supine position, with a waterproof sheet placed under her buttocks. Remember to tilt the woman laterally, if pregnant, to reduce the risk of supine hypotension.

– Wash the hands and put on gloves and a disposable apron.

– Remove any fixings used to secure the catheter to the thigh.

– Using a syringe, withdraw the sterile fluid being used to maintain inflation of the balloon.

– Remove the catheter.

– Make the woman comfortable.

– Empty and measure the amount of urine from the drainage bag.

– Monitor after effects and ensure the woman is able to pass urine.

Breaks in the sealed system between the catheter and drainage bag should be avoided if possible. Any urine samples should be taken by needle aspiration via the sample port on the drainage tubing, in accordance with local policies. Samples should not be taken from the urine bag as it may contain higher concentrations of micro-organisms.

When emptying the drainage bag, the tap should be cleaned before and after use, again according to local procedures. The tap should not touch the sides of the container, be allowed to dip into the urine or touch the floor. The urine should be drained into a container that is later discarded, or thoroughly washed and dried.

Catheter insertion should be performed as an aseptic procedure using sterile gloves and equipment.

Vulval hygiene involving meatal care is an area of debate. The results of trials involving the use of disinfectants such as chlorhexidine or povodine and iodine are not conclusive. Perhaps until more recent research is available, the aim of hygiene care should be to keep the area clean and comfortable by washing and drying with soap and water at least twice a day (Willis, 1996).

The likelihood of infection increases the longer a catheter remains in situ. It should, therefore, be removed as soon as possible.

References

Bayer Diagnostics. *Urinalysis: The Inside Information*. Basingstoke: Bayer Diagnostics, 1996.

Boyle M. *Antenatal Investigations*. Cheshire: Books for Midwives Press, 1994.

Cassidy P. The first stage of labour: physiology and early care. In: Bennett V R, Brown L (eds) *Myles Textbook for Midwives*. Edinburgh: Churchill Livingstone, 1993.

Cook R. Urinalysis: ensuring accurate urine testing. *Nursing Standard*, 1996; 10(46): 49-53.

Enkin M, Keirse M, Renfrew M, Neilson J. (2nd ed) *A Guide to Effective Care in Pregnancy and Childbirth*. Oxford: Oxford University Press, 1996.

Gould D. Keeping on tract. *Nursing Times*, 1994; 90(40): 58-64.

Kennedy A, Brocklehurst J, Lye M. Factors related to problems of long-term catheterisation. *Journal of Advanced Nursing*, 1983; 8: 207-12.

RCN. *Guidelines on Infection Control for Nurses in General Practice*. London: RCN, 1992.

Willis J. Catheters: Urinary tract infections. *Nursing Times*, 1996; 91(35): 48-50.

Tortora G, Anagnostakos N. *Principles of Anatomy and Physiology*. New York: Harper Collins, 1990.

Further reading

Pomfret I. Catheters: design, selection and management. *British Journal of Nursing*. 1996; 5(4): 245-51.

Jamieson E, McCall J, Blythe K, Logan W. *Guidelines for Clinical Nursing Practices*. London: Churchill Livingstone, 1992.

Winn C. Basing catheter care on research principles. *Nursing Standard*, 1996; 10(18): 38-40.

CHAPTER 7

Wound care

As many as 70 per cent of women in the UK are likely to sustain damage to their perineum following childbirth, which is approximately 1000 women per day (Sleep et al, 1984). Other women may have an abdominal wound if their baby was born by caesarean section. A midwife therefore, almost every day has to make decisions about wound care and management.

DEFINITION

A wound can be defined as any bodily injury caused by physical means that disrupts the normal continuity of structures (Solomon et al, 1990).

PHYSIOLOGY

NORMAL WOUND HEALING

Almost immediately that the incision is made by the surgeon or midwife (as in the case of episiotomy), the body initiates an extremely efficient healing process that consists of three stages that overlap each other (Collier, 1996, Strimike et al, 1997). These are:

- The inflammatory (reactive) stage
- The proliferation (regenerative) stage
- The maturation (remodelling) stage

The inflammatory stage lasts for about 3-4 days. Within a few seconds of tissue damage vasoconstriction occurs. Chemicals such as histamine and prostaglandin are released by cells in the injured area. This causes small blood vessels to dilate and become more permeable. That triggers the leakage of plasma and electrolytes into the interstitial spaces, causing swelling. The excess fluid exerts pressure on nerves and other tissues, resulting in pain. The wound at this point is red, hot and painful.

A chemical produced by injured tissue is thought to trigger the release of large numbers of polymorphonuclear leucocytes and macrophages that then appear at the wound site to defend against infection and begin the repair process. They combine to destroy and ingest bacteria and debris.

As blood fills the wound, platelets begin to form a clot. Fibrin, an insoluble protein and essential part of a clot, slowly bridges the edges of the wound. A thin layer of epithelial cells seals the incision and new blood vessels begin to develop.

The proliferation stage is the growth or reproduction of tissue as part of the healing process. It starts from about day 4 and lasts up to three weeks. Macrophage activity stimulates the formation and multiplication of fibroblasts. These migrate along fibrin threads, laying down a ground substance and beginning the synthesis of collagen fibres. Blood cells are trapped in the fibrous network and damaged blood vessels begin to regenerate within the wound margins. The blood vessels branch and join other vessels forming loops. The fragile capillary loops are held within the collagen network. This is known as granulation tissue. During this stage signs of inflammation should subside, although the wound may often remain red.

The maturation stage can last as long as two years but begins between the second and third week (Strimike et al, 1997). The synthesis of granulation tissue and collagen continues, but the collagen strands contract, bringing the edges of the wound closer together and increasing the strength of the tissue. Once the process of contraction is almost complete, re-epithelialisation begins. Epithelial cells from the sides of the wound migrate beneath the scab, eventually meeting and covering the wound. When epithelial cells come in contact with other epithelial cells, their lateral migration is inhibited. Once the wound has been patched, the epithelial cells increase in number to form the strata of the epidermis, beginning to resurface the wounded area (Solomon et al, 1990). Cell division stops when the wound has been repaired. By the time the scab finally falls off, new epidermis is fully formed beneath.

The natural healing process can be achieved by a number of processes. These are:

- Primary intention
- Secondary intention
- Third (tertiary) intention

Healing by primary intention is following a clean surgical incision where the edges of the wound are closely approximated, thus eliminating dead space (Bale and Jones, 1997). Minimal formation of granular tissue occurs, and following healing, only a thin scar remains. All of the phases of wound healing occur but wound contraction only plays a minor role. Epithelium migrate over the suture line to restore tissue integrity.

Healing by secondary intention means the skin edges are deliberately not brought together. This may be as a result of complications from healing by primary intention such as infection. However, it may also have been as a result of a decision made by the midwife, in consultation with the women, to leave a second degree tear unsutured. There is very little evidence available at present to support this decision.

With healing by secondary intention the wound is left to fill with granulation tissue arising from its base. Wound contraction also plays an important role. This can result in dense, fibrous scar tissue with a poor cosmetic result.

There is very little research available to inform the midwife about the advantages and disadvantages of leaving a perineal wound to heal by secondary intention. The information that is available often relates to wounds where there is a large tissue defect such as a pressure sore. Therefore, the information regarding the physiology of wound healing that is available to midwives may not reflect what happens to a small second degree tear that has naturally opposing edges when the women is active and mobile.

Healing by third intention is where a wound, which has not initially been closed surgically, is sutured. It may also occur when a wound breaks down and is then resutured. In the case of infection, a wound may be left open to commence healing by granulation until the underlying problem has resolved. The wound edges are then approximated and healing by primary intention can take place.

FACTORS AFFECTING WOUND HEALING

There are a number factors which the midwife needs to be aware of that may affect wound healing. These include the presence or absence of oxygen, nutrition (especially Vitamin C) and the type of dressing used to cover the wound. However, the most common cause of poor wound healing is probably infection.

In the early stages of wound healing there is an absence of a microcirculation (capillary network) resulting in a low oxygen supply to the tissues. However in this low oxygen environment the macrophages promote new capillary formation resulting in an improved oxygen supply to the tissues. Once the tissue oxygen increases, the healing process continues rapidly. The more vascular the area (such as the perineum) the faster the wound healing.

Anaemia that is caused by the reduction of the number of circulating red blood cells, may have an affect on the tissue oxygenation and therefore the healing process.

Nutrition is becoming important in the understanding of wound healing. Although a significant proportion of the healing process is local and hence occurs despite nutritional inadequacies, where there are deficiencies, wound healing is either delayed or inadequate (Bennett and Moody, 1995). Poor dietary intake is often attributed to the more elderly population but the midwife should consider the woman who is a heavy smoker or perhaps the single, unsupported mother with financial difficulties.

WOUND DRESSINGS

It is usual for a simple dressing to be applied in theatre following a caesarean section. It can be removed about 24 hours post-operatively and no further dressing need be applied. If a small amount of oozing is expected then a semipermeable film may be applied directly to the wound and left in place until the sutures need to be removed. There is much debate however, about the need for dressings at all with sutured wounds (Bale and Jones, 1997).

A wide variety of wound dressings are available. The ideal dressing according to Thomas (1990), should provide an environment at the surface of the wound in which healing may take place at the maximum rate consistent with the production of a healed wound with an acceptable cosmetic appearance. Whitby (1995) believes the principles to remember when assessing the most appropriate dressing to use should:

- Permit gaseous exchange to maintain PO2 and pH at appropriate levels
- Maintain high humidity in the wound as epthelialisation proceeds more rapidly in a moist environment
- Maintain wound temperature close to body core temperature allowing mitosis and phagocytosis to proceed at optimal levels
- Aid removal of dead tissue and bacterial, chemical and physical contaminants
- Be impermeable to bacteria
- Protect healing tissue from disruption by physical forces
- Be non-adherent, non-allergenic and free from contaminants.

CHANGING A DRESSING

In the majority of cases very little is needed to be done by the midwife when dealing with straight forward abdominal wounds that have resulted from a caesarean section. Management is often conservative, applying a dressing in theatre following surgery, which is then removed 24 hours later. A new dressing is not reapplied unless there is a problem. It is important for the midwife to be aware of her own limitations when being asked to undertake a 'complicated' wound dressing. She may need to seek further advice from her nursing colleagues about current techniques and management.

If the wound is clean and little exudate is present, repeated cleansing is contraindicated as it may damage new tissue, decrease the temperature of the wound unnecessarily and remove exudate (Morison, 1989).

If it is necessary to remove the dressing and apply a new one then the following procedure should be followed. The midwife needs also to refer to local policies and guidelines.

If in hospital a dressing trolley is often prepared by washing it clean and putting on the bottom shelf all the equipment that is needed for the procedure. When in the home a clean surface needs to be made available.

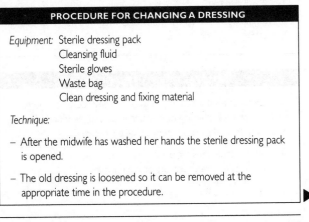

PROCEDURE FOR CHANGING A DRESSING

Equipment: Sterile dressing pack
Cleansing fluid
Sterile gloves
Waste bag
Clean dressing and fixing material

Technique:

– After the midwife has washed her hands the sterile dressing pack is opened.

– The old dressing is loosened so it can be removed at the appropriate time in the procedure.

- The hands should be washed again or cleansed with a bactericidal alcohol rub as they would have become contaminated when handling the outer packets and wound dressing.

- Sterile gloves are then put on.

- The contents of the sterile pack are arranged using the forceps in the pack and lotion is poured into the intended lotion receptacle.

- The dressing is removed in an aseptic manner and disposed of in the waste bag clipped to the side of the dressing trolley.

- The wound is assessed for signs of healing and presence of infection.

- The wound is cleansed with normal saline or another solution which has been prescribed. Each swab is only used once and then disposed of. The wound is then dried, again only using each swab once. If the midwife wears sterile gloves for the cleansing of the wound, it allows for greater sensitivity than forceps and is less likely to traumatise the wound.

- A suitable dressing is applied.

- After the gloves are removed the dressing is secured with non-allergenic tape as required.

- Make sure the woman is comfortable and the dressing secure.

- Wash and dry the trolley again.

- Wash hands with soap and water to prevent the risk of spreading infection.

REMOVAL OF SUTURES AND CLIPS

Non-absorbable sutures or clips should be removed when there is evidence of wound healing or infection in part of the wound. This procedure may take place in hospital or the home.

Equipment: Sterile dressing pack
Stitch cutter, scissors or clip remover
Sterile gloves

Removal of sutures

- After opening the pack in an appropriately clean area, the stitch cutter or scissors are held in the dominant hand and the dissecting forceps in the other hand. The dissecting forceps are used to gently lift the knot of the stitch.

- The knot is cut close to the skin, so that no part of the stitch above the skin surface is pulled under the tissues. This technique helps to reduce the risk of introducing infection.

- The cut stitch is then gently pulled.

- It must be ensured that no piece of the stitch is left in the wound as this may eventually form a wound sinus.

Removal of clips

- The clip remover is held in the dominant hand and the dissecting forceps in the other hand.

- Insert one blade of the clip remover gently under the centre of the clip and the other blade over the top, then gently squeeze the blades together. This causes the clip to 'splay out' and can be removed from the skin.

- The wound may or may not be required to be redressed.

WOUND DRAINS

Wound drains are inserted at the time of surgery to prevent fluid collecting at the wound site. Drains may be stitched in position and attached to a closed circuit bag or portable suction. A portable vacuum suction drain is used to prevent a haematoma forming, by maintaining gentle suction.

CHANGING A VACUUM BOTTLE

Equipment: Primed sterile vacuum bottle
               Cleansing solution

Technique:

- An aseptic technique is followed.

- A sterile vacuum bottle is primed with appropriately cleansed suction apparatus.

- The content of the bottle to be changed is measured and recorded.

- The tube is clamped to prevent air and contamination entering the wound via the drain and the tubing at the connection point is cleansed.

- The bottle is removed.

- The new bottle is attached.

- The clamp is then removed.

- Ensure the vacuum has remained in the bottle.

REMOVAL OF A WOUND DRAIN

Equipment: Sterile dressing pack
               Sterile gloves
               Stitch cutter
               Wound dressing

Technique:

- An aseptic technique is followed.

- The vacuum in the bottle is released.

- If the tubing is stitched, this is first removed.

- The drain is removed gently. If there is any resistance it is helpful to place a gloved hand on the skin next to the tubing to oppose the tugging.

- The drain site should be covered with a sterile dressing.

WOUND ASSESSMENT

Wound assessment is a process that allows the midwife to plan the appropriate management of a woman who has a wound. Factors which need to be taken into account include assessment of the wound as well as of the woman.

In a normal, healthy sutured wound, some degree of inflammation, swelling and redness is to be expected around 2-3 days post-operatively. This indicates that the wound is in the inflammatory phase of healing. If an infection is present, signs and symptoms may include:

- Pyrexia and tachycardia

- Wound beginning to discharge

- The area around the wound becoming red, sore and swollen

- On removal of a suture, pus is discharged

- Partial wound breakdown following removal of sutures.

ASSESSMENT OF PAIN

Pain is an obvious consequence of a surgical wound when related to the physiology of healing. Women have expressed being unprepared for the pain, especially perineal pain, they experienced following the delivery of their baby (Kitzinger and Walters, 1981: Greenshields and Hulme, 1993). Camp and O'Sullivan (1987) also demonstrate that nurses' assessment of pain appears to be very different from that of the patient. The patient is often not believed to be in pain if other signs are absent such as facial expression and raised blood pressure. Nurses decided how much pain a patient had, based on measures other than what the patient said. Therefore, women should be allowed to identify the amount of pain they are experiencing from their own perspective, using pain assessment scores (Way, 1994). Pain assessment should be an integral part of the overall wound assessment.

BODY IMAGE

Body image is the woman's perception of her own appearance and is an integral part of self. Through surgery, whether it be a caesarean section, episiotomy or perineal tear, the woman's body image has been altered or changed. Altered body image can have dramatic negative effects and should be discussed with the woman (Way, 1994). It is recognised that there is a lack of information at present to aid understanding of how a woman perceives her own episiotomy scar. Research in this area is needed to help the midwife approach the concerns of altered body image.

References

Bale S, Jones V. *Wound Care Nursing: A patient-centred approach*. London: Bailliere Tindall, 1997.

Bennett G, Moody M. *Wound Care for Health Professionals*. London: Chapman & Hall, 1995.

Camp L, O'Sullivan P. Comparison of medical, surgical and oncology patients' description of pain and nurses' documentation of pain assessments. *Journal of Advanced Nursing*, 1987; 12(5): 593-8.

Collier M. The principles of optimum wound management. *Nursing Standard*, 1996; 10(43): 47-52.

Greenshields W, Hulme H. *The Perineum in Childbirth. A Survey of Women's experiences and Midwives Practices*. London: National Childbirth Trust, 1993.

Kitzinger S, Walters R. *Some Women's Experiences of Episiotomy*. London: National Childbirth Trust, 1981.

Morison M. Wound cleansing – which solution? *The Professional Nurse*, 1989; 4: 220-5.

Sleep J, Grant J, Elbourne D, Spencer J, Chalmers I. West Berkshire perineal management trial. *British Medical Journal* 1984; 289(6445): 587-90.

Solomon E, Schmidt R, Adranga P. *Human Anatomy & Physiology*. 2nd edition. London: Saunders College Publishing, 1990.

Strimike C, Wojcik J, Stark B. Incision care that really cuts it. *RN*, 1997; July: 22-6.

Thomas S. *Wound Management and Dressing*. London: The Pharmaceutical Press, 1990.

Way S. The Meaning of Episiotomy: A Review of the Historical and Contemporary Literature. Unpublished MSc Dissertation, Surrey University, 1994.

Whitby D. The biology of wound healing. *Surgery*, 1995; 12(2): 25-8.

CHAPTER 8

Care of the immobile woman

There are occasions when the midwife is involved in caring for a woman who is temporarily immobile, either through severe illness or perhaps due to the use of an epidural during labour. There may also be occasions where a woman's physical disability may render her immobile, and so requires the assistance of the midwife, especially in the hospital setting. This chapter seeks to identify how the midwife can assist the woman with her physical comfort, at a time when her immobility may cause a number of medical complications. These complications include such problems as the development of pressure sores, thrombosis or respiratory tract infections and are often referred to in the nursing literature as 'complications of bedrest'.

In most cases, a woman would want to become actively involved in the care of her baby as soon after the birth as possible. This includes those women who have had a caesarean section, who are often out of bed within 12-24 hours of their operation. This early activity and ambulation helps to promote the return of normal physiological activities such as gastrointestinal peristalsis and reduces the incidence of respiratory and circulatory complications.

PRESSURE SORES

A pressure sore or decubitus ulcer is a localised area of skin breakdown resulting from interference with the circulation to the affected tissue(s) (Royle and Walsh, 1992). Blood vessels are squeezed between bony parts of the body and a hard surface, such as a bed or chair. The most consistently cited factors contributing to the development of pressure sores are incontinence, inactivity, restricted mobility, poor nutritional status and mechanical factors such as friction or a shearing force (Sparks, 1993).

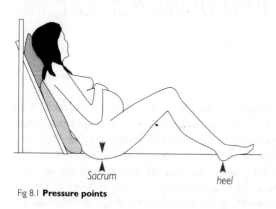

Fig 8.1 **Pressure points**

At a time when a woman has impaired mobility or is immobile, the midwife needs to remember those factors which can contribute to the development of pressure sores. For example, a woman who is experiencing a long labour and has an epidural in situ would certainly have pressure being applied to her sacral area and other bony prominences (Fig 8.1). Her possible inability to move due to the epidural, could result in the circulation to this area being impeded. Moisture may be present from sweating, and if her membranes have ruptured, loss of liquor would also add to the amount of fluid the woman would be sitting in. Shearing forces may exacerbate this if poor lifting techniques are adopted in assisting the woman up and down the bed, especially if she is obese.

Care that would be beneficial to help prevent pressure sores include assessing the woman's risk, preventing her from sitting in sheets soaked with liquor for any length of time, the use of appropriate lifting techniques or lifting aids if necessary and changing her position at least every two hours to relieve pressure of the soft tissues against bone.

THROMBOSIS

There is a large amount of information in the nursing literature about thromboembolic disorders which includes who is at risk, prevention and treatment (THRIFT Consensus Group, 1992, Verstraete, 1997, Wiseman and Cole, 1997). People most at risk :

- Have undergone surgery to the abdomen, pelvis or lower limbs
- Are smokers
- Are obese
- Have a history of deep-vein thrombosis (DVT)

Risk is compounded in those people whose blood has an increased tendency to coagulate such as women who are pregnant. Allotey and Louca (1997) recommend that midwives have a role in the early detection and referral of women suspected of having thromboembolic disorders and provide appropriate health education and advice. Wiseman and Cole (1997) recommend the implementation of research-based and agreed guidelines to reduce the incidence of postoperative DVT. If it remains undetected a DVT can lead to a pulmonary embolus when a fragment of thrombus becomes detached, flows towards the heart, and lodges in a branch of the pulmonary artery to cause infarction beyond.

CAUSES
A number of factors increase the risk of thrombosis, collectively called *Virchow's Triad*. These are:

- Changes in the composition of the blood
- Changes in the rate of blood flow
- Trauma to blood vessels.

CHANGES IN THE COMPOSITION OF THE BLOOD

In pregnancy, blood constituents such as Fibrinogen, Factor VII, Factor X, and platelets are all increased, leading to a change in the coagulation time from 12 to 8 minutes. As the capacity for clotting is increased, there is a resultant higher risk of thrombosis and embolism. These changes in coagulation factors can be detected from about the third month of pregnancy and are influenced by rising oestrogen levels and alterations in the metabolism of clotting factors by the liver.

CHANGES IN RATE OF FLOW

During pregnancy, as the gravid uterus grows, there is increased pressure on the pelvic veins, reducing circulatory blood flow, especially affecting the legs. Bed rest, for whatever reason, will reduce circulatory blood flow even further, especially venous return from the legs. This is because muscle activity in the calf enhances blood flow and venous return, so becomes reduced during periods of inactivity.

TRAUMA TO BLOOD VESSELS

This can result from surgery, hypertensive disease or local blood-borne infection that could follow any birth but especially caesarean section. The Report on the Confidential Enquiry into Maternal Deaths (Department of Health, 1996) highlighted that 13 of the 17 maternal deaths from thromboembolism in the puerperium had occurred in women delivered by caesarean section. The Royal College of Obstetrics and Gynaecology Working Party (RCOG, 1995) devised a stratified risk assessment profile recommending a range of prophylactic treatment for women undergoing caesarean operations. This includes categorising women as low, moderate or high risk from developing a thromboembolism. Criteria identifying which women fit into which category is listed with the appropriate management for each. Women classified as high risk should receive prophylactic heparin, and leg stockings are beneficial. The prophylactic heparin is recommended until the 5th day or until fully mobile if sooner.

Colditz et al (1986) suggests the literature is clear about the use of full length anti-embolic stockings reducing the risk of people developing DVT. These stockings provide degrees of external compression which enhances blood flow and venous return by putting external pressure on vein walls. This brings the vascular cusps into contact with one another, preventing pooling and increasing blood-flow velocity. All randomised studies reporting the efficacy of these stockings have used the same brand – TED (Drug and Therapeutic Bulletin, 1992). This brand of stocking is apparently the only one that has been supported by clinical trials and has an educational support programme to enhance its use (Wiseman and Cole, 1997).

Deep breathing and leg exercises should be taught whilst the woman is in bed and she should be encouraged to do them frequently to reduce the risks of thromboembolic disorders, which are higher following an operative delivery (Department of Health, 1996). Leg exercises can be commenced 8-12 hours after surgery and done every 2-3 hours until the woman is mobile. The exercises include alternating active flexion and extension of the toes and dorsal and plantar flexion of the feet. This encourages venous return from the legs. Early ambulation also decreases the frequency of DVT in the puerperium.

RESPIRATORY TRACT INFECTION

Impaired respiratory function may lead to a respiratory tract infection and could occur following a caesarean section. This is because pain from the abdominal wound may prevent adequate expansion of the lungs. The risk of a respiratory tract infection could be further compounded if the woman is a smoker or if she has had a general anaesthetic.

Prevention of post-operative respiratory complications can be helped by pre-operative preparation. However this is only possible with a woman who is having a planned caesarean section, allowing the midwife to explain to the woman what will happen, what to expect and even practice some of the exercises taught before the operation. The exercises taught would involve deep breathing, assisting maximal lung expansion.

Deep breathing exercises resulting in sustained maximal inspiration should carried out post-operatively several times each hour. The woman is helped into a position to allow for maximum chest expansion (such as sitting up) and is encouraged to take a deep breath, hold for about 3-5 seconds and then breathe out slowly (Royle and Walsh, 1992).

If the woman needs to cough, she should bend her knees and support her wound with a pillow or hands whilst leaning forward. This will prevent undue strain on the sutures, increase the woman's confidence and reduce pain. A sitting position is best for both activities. It is important that the woman's level of pain is first assessed and medication given to alleviate the pain.

Midwives should work in partnership with the physiotherapist with any woman they may be concerned about.

PERSONAL HYGIENE CARE

When a woman is unable to mobilise because of ill health or having undergone surgery then at some point she may need assistance with washing in bed. If the woman is critically ill then she may be completely dependent on the midwife for her personal hygiene care, which may include, what is commonly referred to in the nursing textbooks, as a blanket bath.

PROCEDURE FOR A BLANKET BATH

Equipment:	Personal toiletry items
	Two towels
	Clean clothes
	Sanitary towels and pants
	Washing bowl
	Hair care items

▶

Technique:

- The basic procedure should be explained to the woman first (if she is conscious and able to respond) as she may wish to be bathed by a relative, or request that her husband is not present, especially when the vulval area needs cleansing (Schott and Henley, 1996).

- It is helpful if two people are able to assist with bathing the woman in bed, to help with positioning the woman during the procedure.

- Warmth is important, so the area should be free from draughts, curtains drawn, doors closed and screens used where necessary.

- All the equipment and toiletry items should be within reach during the procedure.

- As much as possible the woman should be encouraged to attend to her own needs.

- Always ask the woman at each stage what she would like. Some women may like to use soap, others do not, some use deodorant, talc etc.

- Throughout the bath it is important to talk to the woman as it is an ideal opportunity to chat and to give information (Way, 1996).

- Care needs to be taken with wound dressings as well as intravenous infusion sites.

- The vulval area should be left to last. If this is not possible the water needs to be changed and the bowl cleaned.

MANUAL HANDLING ISSUES

Back injury is the most common single hazard for midwives and nurses. Midwives are at risk due to the fact that a lot of their time can be spent stooping or bending, for a variety of reasons such as helping a woman to breast feed, supporting women birthing their babies in alternative positions and care of high dependency women (Dimond, 1994). The lack of published research on work-related back pain in midwifery indicates that this area does not seem to have received the attention it deserves (Hignett, 1996).

In 1992, legislation was introduced recommending the use of an ergonomic approach to the risk management of health and safety. One specific area of guidance was manual handling operations (Manual handling, 1992). Croner Publications Ltd (1997) define 'Manual handling operations' as 'any transporting or supporting of a load (including lifting, putting down, pushing, pulling, carrying or moving thereof by hand or by bodily force)'. The definition of load includes the handling of a person, so that the actions of moving a woman in a hospital constitutes a manual handling operation.

THE SHOULDER LIFT (Darby, 1993; Teaching Support and Media Services 1994)

Technique:

- The height of the bed is first adjusted so it is positioned halfway between the hips and knees of the midwives performing the lift.

- The brakes need to be applied and the midwives performing the lift stand either side of the bed.

- The leading foot should face the moving direction that the lift is to take place.

- The hips and knees are bent, with the back remaining in its natural curves.

- The midwives position their near-side shoulders next to the chest wall of the woman, under her axilla, while the woman places her arms down the midwives' backs.

- The handling sling is placed high under the woman's thighs and the midwives hold the sling.

- The other hand is placed on the bed behind the woman to support her trunk. The elbows are flexed ready to take the weight.

- The 'leading' midwife gives the 'agreed' orders.

- Slowly the trailing leg and elbow is straightened and the woman is lifted clear of the bed.

- The woman is then lowered to the bed as the midwives bend the leading leg and supporting elbow.

- The woman should only be moved a short distance at a time.

CORE SKILLS FOR CARING AND ASSESSMENT

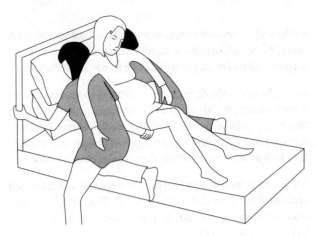

Fig 8.2 **Shoulder lift**

When lifting a load it is important to remember to maintain the natural curves in the back, of which there are 3; the hollow at the neck and lower back and the outward curve in between (Teaching Support and Media Services, 1994). The load should be kept close to the body and there should be a stable base of support, that is the feet should be firmly positioned flat on a firm base.

Within midwifery, moving or repositioning a woman in bed whose mobility may be temporarily limited, is probably the most common reason to move a heavy load. To some extent, each woman's mobility will be determined by her own physical capabilities. The woman should be given as much opportunity as possible to move independently. She should only be helped to the extent that she is unable to move freely without assistance.

If the decision has been made to reposition a woman in the bed and it requires a lift, then probably the most appropriate lift is the shoulder lift. Local policies should be used to guide the decision and procedure.

Before undertaking the lift, the task and load, environment and capabilities are all assessed. It is determined how much the woman can do for herself; how heavy the woman is and should a mechanical aid be used to help with the lift; is there enough room around the bedside to perform the lift safely and that the floor is not slippery; and finally are you the midwife able to undertake the lift?

Each individual midwife has a responsibility to ensure that they are trained, competent and able to assess situations to the best of their abilities. A midwife should never lift a woman unless absolutely necessary and alternative measures should always be considered first, such as the woman helping herself as much as possible.

If a lift is necessary then everyone involved should know and understand the plan of lifting and handling. There must be enough space to lift, making sure that there are no obstacles in the way and that the floor is not slippery.

References

Allotey J, Louca O. Thromboembolic disorders: treatment and diagnosis. *British Journal of Midwifery*, 1997; 5(2): 75-9.

Colditz G, Tuden R, Oster G. Rates of venous thrombosis after general surgery: combined results of randomised clinical trials. *The Lancet*, 1986; 2: 143-6.

Croner Publications Ltd. *Health and Safety at Work*. London: Croner, 1997.

Darby S. Lifting and handling patients. In: *The Handbook for Hospital Care Assistants and Support Workers*. Ed Swiatczak L, Benson S. London: Hawker Publications Ltd, 1993.

Department of Health. *Report on Confidential Enquiries into Maternal Deaths in the United Kingdom 1991-1993*. London: HMSO, 1996.

Dimond B. The midwife and risk management at work. *Modern Midwife*, 1994; 4(4): 36-7.

Drug and Therapeutics Bulletin. Preventing and treating deep-vein thrombosis. *Drug and therapeutics Bulletin*, 1992; 30: 3.

Hignett S. Manual handling risks in midwifery: identification of risk factors. *British Journal of Midwifery*, 1996; 4(11): 590-6.

Manual Handling. *Manual Handling Operations Regulations 1992 Guidance of Regulations L23*. London: HSE Books, 1992.

Royal College of Obstetricians and Gynaecology. *RCOG Working party on Prophylaxis Against Thromboembolism in Gynaecology and Obstetrics*. London: RCOG, 1995.

Royle J, Walsh M. *Watson's Medical-Surgical Nursing and Related Physiology*. London: Bailliere Tindall, 1992.

Schott J, Henley A. *Culture, Religion and Childbearing in a Multiracial Society*. London: Butterworth Heinemann, 1996.

Sparks S. Clinical validation of pressure ulcer risk factors. *Ostomy/Wound Management*, 1993; 24(4): 40-50.

Teaching Support and Media Services. *Straight Forward Back Care for Nurses*. Southampton: University of Southampton, 1994.

Thromboembolic Risk Factors (THRIFT) Consensus Group. The report of the national confidential enquiry into perioperative deaths 1991/92. *British Medical Journal*, 1992; 305(6853): 567-74.

Verstraete M. Prophylaxis of venous thromboembolism. *British Medical Journal*, 1997; 314(7074): 123-5.

Way S. Post-delivery personal hygiene care. *British Journal of Midwifery*, 1996; 4(6): 633-6.

Wiseman C, Cole A. Guidelines for preventing thromboembolism. *Professional Nurse*, 1997; 12(7): 485-7.